Multiple Sclerosis: psychological and social aspects

Multiple Sclerosis: psychological and social aspects

Edited by

Aart F Simons

Consultant Psychologist, Queensland Multiple Sclerosis Society, Australia

William Heinemann Medical Books
London

1984

First published 1984
by William Heinemann Medical Books Ltd,
23 Bedford Square,
London WC1B 3HH

ISBN 0–433–30295–X

Typeset by Inforum Ltd, Portsmouth
Printed in Great Britain by
Biddles Ltd, Guildford

Contents

Preface

This book is intended to fill what I have felt to be a gap in the literature on multiple sclerosis. It is an international book on the psychological and social aspects of MS for all those who work in the field of MS care, who study in this area and for those people with MS who wish to go beyond some of the pamphlets handed out to them on diagnosis.

I hope that in this book, most of the issues that concern those working in the field are at least raised. Many authors contributed to this book from many countries around the world. If all papers submitted had been included, the size of the book would have trebled and it would have become too cumbersome. It was a difficult task to decide which articles to leave out, and the final version represents a personal choice of subjects and material.

I would like to give some brief explanation of my purpose and of the way I hope the book will be used. Above all, it is not meant to be read from one chapter to the next. Rather, it is intended as a resource— as a place to find opinions which can be challenged and discussed. Each chapter, therefore, can be read on its own and of necessity duplicates some of the facts in other chapters. The basic reason for this is that the psychosocial reactions and consequences of MS cannot be easily separated, as each reaction can provoke another consequence. I have not provided a common terminology for all chapters. Therefore, one author may use the word patient, whereas others use descriptions such as sufferers or people with multiple sclerosis.

I have given my biased feelings from the point of view of aiding the adaptation process about the terminology in Chapter 1 and hope that that is provocative enough to encourage thought.

In the first chapter, I have tried to suggest ways in which support can be given to people with MS and their families. By making readers aware of the various conflicts that have to be faced as well as of the contradictory messages in the rehabilitation setting, it may help those working in the area to introduce new concepts in their care for those suffering from MS and their families.

The next two chapters deal with specific reactions two people have had towards MS and their own special psychosocial triumphs over the disease process. Both are presently living around MS, recognising all the good things that life has brought them as well.

Chapter 4 is probably most helpful for doctors who have to impart the diagnosis of MS. Specific here is the advice to communicate not only the facts but, while doing this, to be aware of the emotional needs of the newly diagnosed person.

Chapter 5 focuses not just on the personal shock of being diagnosed, but on the fact that it involves the family, close and far, and the community in the sense of work and friends. Although the family has changed its role over the years, it is still the important primary provider of help and support.

Chapter 6 looks at the general interaction between neurological factors and inter- and intrapersonal factors which govern the way people cope with sexual alterations in their lives due to MS. It clearly shows that the recognition of this interaction is the most important element in recognising and dealing with the sexual implications of MS.

Chapter 7 deals with emotional reactions to MS and finds that endogenous depression, as a direct consequence of cerebral damage (due to MS), is commonly due to changes in the limbic system and the frontal lobe. Such damage frequently leads to endogenous depression and, less frequently, mania.

Chapter 8 looks further into the frontal-lobe function and the authors suggest that alteration of cognitive ability and affective function is due to the deterioration of this lobe rather than to affective reaction to the disease.

Chapter 9 indicates that MS generally attracts stigma and that technological and sociological barriers prevent the integration of MS-disabled and those with other disabilities. The effect of disability on the non-disabled is discussed, and reported as having an adverse effect on them. This makes resolution essential for both able and disabled in order for them to interact less stressfully. This chapter indicates that the MS-disabled themselves are the best advocates of their needs, and suggests that MS societies should perhaps be more composed *of* MS-disabled people rather than *for* MS disabled people.

Chapter 10 shows the importance of recreation and leisure for those disabled with MS. It makes a clear point that one should encourage MS-disabled people to take risks and that we should not let our own fears and limited imagination prevent them from participating and perhaps even failing to achieve in certain areas.

Chapter 11 points out that rehabilitation is still seen as most effective by people with MS when it helps them to approximate, as closely as possible, to society's image of the ideal person. The conflict that this creates may well point in the direction of a changed rehabilitation objective.

I have used individual chapters for teaching purposes and each chapter can, more or less, be used on its own. Most have their own bibliographies which provide a chance to assess the evidence.

ACKNOWLEDGEMENTS

Producing the book has for me been hard labour and I would like to thank Fran Simons, Vic Barnes and Rex Newsome for their criticism and advice. Hank Dassel's encouragement and the support of the IFMSS were also greatly appreciated.

I should also like to thank all those people with MS I have spoken to around the world. The book is for them!

Problems of Providing Support for People with Multiple Sclerosis and their Families

Aart Simons is a psychologist in private practice in Brisbane, Australia; a consultant psychologist with the Queensland Multiple Sclerosis Society; and permanent guest lecturer on MS to The Royal Nursing School in Brisbane.

In this chapter he considers the effects of information on the responses of people with MS and how this information affects their behaviour and expectations. He looks at the processes involved from health to illness, disability to rehabilitation, and the support necessary and problems encountered during these stages. The emphasis of the chapter is on marital relationships, although other affected relationships are explored briefly, and possible aspects of assistance for the MS sufferers and their families discussed.

The Oxford Dictionary defines the word 'support' as meaning 'to give strength to' or 'to encourage'. Giving strength to the person with MS, his family, relatives and others of importance in the light of what is generally said about MS is a clear necessity. However, how does one give strength to others, particularly to those who are in many ways different from ourselves, different in expectations of life and fears about the future, and who have just experienced a general reduction in the quality of their lives? Empathy, perhaps, is an important component in giving strength to a person with MS. The ability to put oneself in the other person's shoes, thereby achieving understanding of such a person, makes emotional communication possible and helps in the achievement of meaningful adaptational responses.

An even more important aspect of giving strength to the person with MS is the help a psychologist or someone else trained in interpersonal skills can give in enabling such a person to get to know himself more and, as a result, open the possibility of growth. As part of this process, I frequently ask people with MS to write out or say their answers to the following.

1. What MS is to them.
2. What MS is not.
3. What they like about MS.
4. What they do not like about it.
5. What they have given up that they like, because of MS.
6. What other things they can do, having MS.

Such an approach allows a person to discover new meaning in what he is doing and what he might want to do. Even if he makes a decision to do nothing new, or to make no changes, he will still have a better feeling of *what* he is doing and *who* he is. Such feelings can then be explored and can provide the support needed to take the next step: to explore where he might want to go when he is ready to make the move.

However, such a step is frequently difficult to make, in that many persons with MS think that it closes the door on many, if not all, directions of their lives. Such thoughts are not infrequently due to the literature that is handed out to people on diagnosis, their own feelings about disability, as well as the feelings of their families and friends and the, at times quite nihilistic, attitude of society in general toward disability.

A quick overview of research in the psychosocial area should, in fact, convince most of us that MS must be a tremendous burden on people diagnosed with the disease and those who live with them. Of course, it does not only convince us, but also the MS sufferers themselves, and hence develops an expectation set which frequently leads to symptoms which may have little to do with MS. For example, preparatory depression is found in persons with MS. This is a depression that does not occur as a result of a past loss, but takes into account impending losses. Looking at the variety of losses over and above the possible physical ones the MS person feels he might have to face as a result of reading the literature that is handed to him, or from talking to others who have read the research, it becomes clear that support should be given quickly to alleviate these preparatory aspects of anxiety and depression, by explaining the meaning of such research. Research has, for example, illuminated many problem areas in relation to MS which include:

1. sexual problems;[1]
2. aggressive behaviour;[2]
3. personality changes;[3]

4. anxiety;[4]
5. poor family relationships in general;[5,6]
6. mental deterioration;[7]
7. depression/euphoria;[8]
8. suicide risk;[9]
9. poor job placement;[10]
10. self-concept changes;[11]
11. society's negative reaction to disability.[12]

Research here is usually in survey form and states that x% of the surveyed population experienced this or that problem at such and such a level of statistical significance when compared to the total normal population. These surveys do help in the respect that they alert many of the helping professions to the fact that MS causes many people to suffer in some or all of these areas. The difficulty, however, lies in the fact that the MS population is not a strictly confined group in the sense of population group divisions based on age, sex, profession and social status, since MS is found in all these groups. It is recognised that if a person is young or old, male or female, or in needy circumstances, for example, this may influence the extent of each problem as well as that person's needs as regards rehabilitation requirements and social integration. For example, it is evident that males with MS tend to suffer more psychologically and socially than do females with MS. This is because the disease process is incongruent with the cultural role of men. For example, in many Western societies the role of women is still mainly seen as concerned with household responsibilities and the rearing of children. This role normally entails social isolation. Disability resulting from MS can result in confinement to the home and severence from community ties. An American comparison of psychological stress symptom rates between housewives and unemployed men suggested that similar high rates of stress in the two groups may be related to restriction to the home.[13] Isolation from social contacts is, in fact, the single most important consequence of 'housewifery'. Many women in this role, however, have already tended to develop some coping strategies against this stress, whereas men, through unemployment and/or disability, are suddenly forced into isolation with no coping strategies at all and, in the case of disability, even fewer outlets than the average housewife or unemployed man. Also, women are not looked down upon if they stay at home, whereas men are socially devalued as a result of staying at home, which introduces even more stress.

Males also tend to suffer more than females in that they face a further handicap in dealing with MS because social constraints curb their emotional expressivity. When compared with females, this relative lack of emotional outlet tends to cause different adaptational processes for each sex.

It should also be understood that conclusions drawn from many studies do not help any of us to understand the individual faced with MS, and that in fact, no neat model of care can be given because of the wide variety of factors that impinge on each person with MS, which tends to produce different reactions and therefore different needs and expectations of care and support.

The list of possible symptoms of MS, both physical and psychological, and the variety of reactions to MS researched, frighten many, in particular those newly diagnosed people, as many feel they, of necessity, will get all these symptoms and reactions as they are stated to be a part of the disease process of MS. Such thinking can cause the already mentioned preparatory anxiety and depression. The person with MS is also made aware through the literature of the lack of certainty in MS prognosis and the fact that he is not expected to develop all these symptoms. It is, however, this lack of certainty that causes many of the worst reactions through the fear of getting *all* the possible symptoms. Such a fear can come to a head when a newly diagnosed person is first brought into contact with an MS centre where he sees in those around him the range of symptoms the disease can produce. He then tends to watch his fellow sufferers anxiously and adds their symptoms to the imagined list of symptoms he feels he will develop. The lack of certainty in MS prognosis, however, can also be used in a positive sense. Lowry (see Chapter 3), a Canadian with MS, stated, in this regard, that 'the kindest comment the doctors could make was that they could not even guess what the future held for me'. Such a comment is also far more honest and acceptable to the person with MS than comments which are given at times to such people when they state their fears about the type of symptoms they might develop. People with MS have frequently told me that after having stated their fears, even to professionals, they were often told by professionals that they were not likely to develop further symptoms — a comment obviously given as a means to alleviate anxiety in them. However, such a comment was generally made after the person with MS had been told that comparatively little is known about the disease and that no control over its progress can be established. The contradiction between 'no control' and 'not likely to develop' is picked up by the person with MS, who tends to feel conned, at best, and loses faith in the professional at worst. Such a loss of faith can result in hostile non-cooperative behaviour which could have been easily avoided.

To begin to support a person with MS, one needs therefore to become aware of at least some of the pressures and fears with which he is faced, not only through the uncertainty and unpredictability of the disease process, but also through the introduction of information on the disease and the way he tends to read it. Furthermore, because of the variety of reactions to the disease as a result of many factors, including the person's previous coping style, personality characteristics, intelligence and other factors, it is important to gather as much information as possible about the person with MS and, in particular, to understand the process in which he was transformed from a healthy person into a person with disability. Such information allows for the giving of more effective support through the setting of individual programmes which utilise this background information.

THE PROCESS FROM HEALTH TO ILLNESS

Here again, from individual psychotherapy and group therapy with MS sufferers, the various ways in which people suffering with MS have gone from one stage to the other become apparent.

1. There are those who, immediately after the appearance of abnormal but not severe and incapacitating symptoms, define the symptoms as potential illness and consult a physician for diagnosis and care. This group in particular appears to have great faith in the curative aspect of medicine, tends to be authority oriented and feels greatly disillusioned with the role of medicine once the 'no cure' statement of MS has been pronounced. However, despite this disillusionment, this group of people with MS still entertains the authority role of medicine and is best helped by prescribing, rather than suggesting, physical and psychological treatment, with a medical doctor seen as the all-important person in charge.

2. Then there are those who consult a doctor only after self-determined or lay-determined treatment has failed to ameliorate their condition and their lay consultants finally refer them to a doctor, or after their condition has become severe and visible. Those in this group selectively or temporarily omit or curtail certain activities or tasks they feel are not essential or even definitely detrimental to their state of health. It seems that the relinquishing of task activities does not have to be legitimised by a doctor, but depends on the degree of acceptance and support this decision receives from significant others. People in this group present now as they did in the early stages of feeling ill, as self-reliant and as placing more faith in the self, and should be allowed and encouraged to be more active in the treatment process by participating

in goal setting. Family involvement in this group is imperative. Within a nursing-home-type setting, these people also respond better if they can somehow retain some self-direction within the institutionalised framework.

3. Then there are those who, despite awareness of abnormal symptoms which they at times define as illness and at times not, are unwilling to assume the sick role and forfeit their social role. Mostly, these are individuals who could not afford to fall sick or who could not afford to take the time. They will only give in to illness when it becomes so severe that it drastically interferes with the performance of various social roles which they deem to be crucial in their lives. This group presently tends to show the most psychological symptoms in that the sick role, once taken on, tends to be seen as a personal failure, and social withdrawal is common once the sick role is assumed to be permanent. This group appears to be best helped by reinforcing the concept that a person with MS, although suffering from a disease, is not ill in the traditional sense of the word. Here, for example, the following conceptualisation of how we generally tend to view the sick role is given. A person in the sick role should:

a. be exempted from social responsibilities (after legitimisation of symptoms by a doctor);
b. not be expected to take care of himself;
c. want to get well;
d. seek medical advice and co-operate with medical experts.

However, once the sickness has been medically diagnosed as MS, in other words as an incurable, disabling disease and no longer an illness, the person is then in fact expected to behave in a totally different way from that which was initially expected from him when he assumed the sick role.

THE PROCESS FROM ILLNESS TO DISABILITY

The label of 'sickness', although it can imply severity, also implies a temporary condition which can, through some kind of intervention, usually medical, be made to disappear. It is the label of disability only that carries a connotation of irreversibility, regardless of the degree of severity of the condition. Because of this distinctive connotation, the person with MS tends to be less willing to accept it as a label and, in fact, some people disabled by MS never accept it, even when they have had to sacrifice reality in order to avoid the negative effects of its stigma. Of course, here too, a person's significant others, such as the family, play an important role in influencing him either to accept or to reject the label of disability.

Sometimes, however, relatives or family may define the person with MS in a way that he himself is never willing to accept. In current research on family reactions to MS,[5] there is some evidence coming to the fore that, in the case of MS, the nature of the husband/wife relationship prior to the onset of the disabling symptoms determines whether the non-affected spouse will accept the label of MS and permanent disability or resist this label, even at the expense of reality. For example, it was found that spouses highly satisfied with their marriages before the onset of MS, tended to fight the label of physical illness longer, which to them is a permanent and irreversible label. However, spouses who were dissatisfied with their marriages prior to the onset of MS, showed some eagerness in accepting the permanent label of physical illness. These spouses seemed to welcome a serious and irreversible disability, probably because it reinforced the already present desire to disassociate themselves from the now stigmatised spouse. This disassociation frequently progressed from an emotional break to a break in the marital relationship, particularly through the process of alienation by which the MS-disabled spouse was denied the chance of reintegration within the family. It was also found that wives of some MS-disabled men who had always wished to work tended to encourage their husbands' dependency and thereby fostered their inability to work in order to have the opportunity of assuming the vocational breadwinner role themselves, and that also middle-aged disabled husbands tended to accept this role rearrangement better than did younger people. Clearly, the significant others play an important role in the acceptance or rejection of the label of disability.

THE PROCESS FROM DISABILITY TO REHABILITATION— THE DISABLED ROLE

From the time that MS leaves residuals or, indeed, gets worse, rehabilitation personnel tend to assign the disabled role to the individual whether he wishes to assume it or not. The way rehabilitation personnel conceptualise the disabled role is based on the way they wish the MS-disabled to behave. This may vary from one MS centre to another, but there are indications that rehabilitation personnel in general would seem to like the disabled person to behave as follows.

1. *He should accept disability and start learning how to live with it.* One

basic difficulty here, however, appears again and again in individual therapy with people who have MS— they are unwilling to accept the fact that medical science can do nothing for them in terms of curing. This is due to a number of factors; partially because psychologically the person with MS cannot accept the fact that he will remain disabled, and also because different doctors have been consulted but have not been entirely in agreement as to the prognosis due to the nature of MS. This ambiguity encourages the MS person's desire to cease being disabled altogether. Anybody, therefore, who offers the promise of diminishing the degree of disability will be consulted in order that the painful acceptance of permanent disability can be postponed indefinitely. In this phase, the MS person continues going from doctor to doctor, to osteopath, chiropractor, and people who are willing to promise unrealistic, miraculous results. This non-acceptance of the disabled role by the MS person should therefore not be seen as an indication that such a person is mentally ill and is denying reality; he might just be fighting a self-concept change that he feels may not be necessary if there is the promise of a cure still around.

2. *The person with MS is also expected to be motivated to do better* and his motivation must be geared towards effective utilisation of remaining abilities in order to resume as many of his normal social roles as possible. It appears, in fact, that there is an assumption that the MS-disabled person, regardless of his level of disability, is always interested and willing to master his environment and to go on struggling with life, meeting its requirements. Many of those who do not fit this assumption are considered not to be interested, to be lazy, to be mentally ill, and are at times dismissed from certain parts of the rehabilitation programme. People with MS who do attempt to go on struggling with life, particularly by continued social activities and social interaction, meet with much conflict within themselves and with those able-bodied people around them. On the one hand, self-reliance, independence and autonomy are highly valued and emphasised by society. However, disabled persons in general seem to be subjected to societal pressures; pressures directing them towards assuming a helpless handicapped role, at least when they interact socially with non-disabled. Presumably, this negative pressure exists because the total assumption of the handicapped role facilitates interaction for the non-disabled who can then, usually on the basis of stereotypic impressions, rather easily assess the limits and restrictions which the disability imposes upon the mode of interaction. The results of group therapy seem to indicate that because of this normative ambiguity concerning their expected behaviour, social contacts with the non-disabled are avoided or can go to either of two extremes—excessive

normalisation or excessive handicapping—none of these reactions helping the person with MS to maintain his motivation.

The disabled role assigned to the MS person can then generate conflict, ambiguity and associated feelings of anxiety, feelings of indecision and loss of motivation.

3. At MS rehabilitation centres, it is generally expected that *the person with MS must be actively involved in his rehabilitation* and, in essence, be an agent of change rather than a passive object in the hands of the rehabilitation team. He must not only comply with suggestions and co-operate with team members' efforts but also innovate and improvise new ways to circumvent his physical restrictions. Here again, it is essential to know the social psychological background of the person with MS. This is because sociological research suggests that middle-class disabled people may conform more closely to this role expectation because they have been accustomed to exercises that require a certain degree of mastery over their lives. Working-class disabled people, on the other hand, socialised to comply and follow orders and not be self-reliant, particularly those whose prevalent mode of behaviour is of passive compliance, may have difficulty fulfilling this expectation.[14] Here again then, one can help the MS-disabled person in a variety of ways. In this case, firstly, by taking the social-class differences into account in the treatment programme and, secondly, by becoming aware of some of the confusing messages that some people with MS receive on entering a rehabilitation centre. Take for example the situation in which people arriving at the rehabilitation centre may, and often do, perceive it as a hospital where passive compliance is required and rewarded. Despite the fact that the difference between the rehabilitation setting and that of a hospital has usually been briefly explained, they may still be rewarded for passive compliance. Short or inadequate explanations as well as the contradictory message on passivity and active involvement may lead to such people failing to become socialised into the acceptable rehabilitation role. Further confusion results from a failure to point out the difference between the role of a rehabilitant and that of a sick person. Such confusion begins on entry to the centre, when they are called patients, with the connotation of the sick role, and yet are expected to do all the things that are expected of a rehabilitant. This might be seen by some as 'nit picking', but words are very important and I feel that once a person has been accepted in a rehabilitation setting, the word 'patient' should no longer be applied to him as it makes the adaptation process to the disabled role with its different connotations very difficult to achieve. In this regard, one centre in Brisbane calls the consumers of its services 'rehabilitatees'. Perhaps this word does not sit right with many, but at

least it is an attempt to make the adaptation process less stressful, by allowing an easier transition from the sick role to the disabled role.

So far, the surface has only been scratched of what is an important aspect of supporting people with MS, particularly from a psychosocial point of view. That is, that there is no such person as an MS person, an MS personality, that one cannot tar all people with MS with the same brush. One needs in fact to become very much aware of the individual differences, not only in symptoms of MS but of the person's reactions to these symptoms, his background, his personality, his general coping styles, his family supports, his family rejections, society's generally negative approaches to disability and the confused messages in the rehabilitation process.

Some more specific types of supporting interventions that can be made for specific symptoms where they are expressed in the person with MS will now be considered. Again, of necessity, only some will be described, although many symptoms need supporting interventions. Again, the suggested interventions are not applicable to all people with MS, but should be seen as a helpful guide in offering solutions to some.

MANAGEMENT OF SEXUAL DIFFICULTIES

While many of the sexual symptoms researched can, and do, arise as a direct consequence of nerve damage associated with the disease, they can also arise indirectly as a result of psychological or relational reactions to MS. However, it is quite often difficult to ascertain which of the symptoms are a result of neurological damage and which are a result of psychological or relational reactions to MS. In Chapter 6 Barrett looks at some methods currently available for distinguishing between organic and psychogenic sexual dysfunction, but clearly states that these methods should be approached with cautious optimism in relation to people with MS, particularly as the distinctions can be misleading in a variable condition such as MS.

Looking at social research in the sexual area, one should be particularly careful when a person with MS comes up with sexual problems. Remember that the research is again based on percentages and we should never say 'It is part of MS and you will have to learn to live with it'. In fact, MS does not, and therefore should not, spell an end to sexual pleasure and satisfaction. Knowledge of the sexual implications of the disease— and here one can study articles by Barrett[1] and Burnfield[15]— coupled with a willingness on behalf of the partners to experiment and to communicate openly about the problems, can help people cope with the changes in their sexual responses and relationships. Sex, however, is a topic that people with MS and perhaps other disabilities prefer not to talk about for a variety of reasons. It has in fact been reported by some group therapists that when the topic of sexual adjustment was raised within the group and set as a topic to be discussed at the next session, less than 50% of the group attended that session.[2] However, by having sexual information available and encouraging discussions about sexual concerns, psychologists, doctors and social workers can diffuse minor problems before they develop into larger relationship-threatening crises. Perhaps also, rather than discussing this at a group session, problems might be easier discussed in a more private one-to-one situation.

On a relationship basis, the loss of libido and the specific physical and psychological symptoms which affect the person with MS may lead the non-affected spouse, whose libido has not changed and who is physically capable of unchanged sexual activity, quite often to feel more distressed than the person with MS. The non-affected partner, it has been found in ongoing research,[5] may also think that the person with MS is no longer interested in the physical aspects of the relationship and may look for these outside the marriage. Here again then, more information should be given to the non-affected spouse as well as to the affected one in order to induce a willingness to experiment and, particularly, to communicate openly about their feelings which can then help them cope *within* the relationship with changes in sexual responses and needs.

MANAGEMENT OF ANGER AND AGGRESSION IN GENERAL

Aggression and anger have been reported frequently in the literature on MS. Both are frequently related to frontal-lobe damage, but, in my opinion, also frequently arise out of frustration of basic needs. These needs may include the need to be loved, the need to explore, and the need for expressing one's individuality. The latter in particular is commonly blocked in a hospital setting. In contrast to the stage of denial which has quite often been mentioned as one of the earliest stages in the reaction to diagnosis, the state of anger appears to be very difficult to cope with from the point of view of the person with MS, his family and staff. The reason for this is that anger is frequently displaced in all directions, projected onto the environment at times almost randomly. Comments such as 'Doctors are just no good'; 'They don't know what we require', and 'They don't know what diets to prescribe'; 'We are kept too long in the hospital'; and 'Our wishes are not respected in regard to special privileges', are indicative of this anger. Nurses in particular appear to be a frequent target of anger. However, visiting family and friends can also become a target and are received with little cheerfulness and anticipation during this stage, which makes the encounter a painful event. As a result, such visitors tend to avoid future visits, which only increases the discomfort of the person with MS and produces further anger and guilt feelings. Beside frontal-lobe damage and blocked needs, where else does this anger come from? Well, perhaps we too would be angry if our life's activities were interrupted so prematurely, if we were reminded frequently that we cannot even stand on our own two feet any more, while others busily rush around us; also, that people order unpleasant tests or prolonged hospitalisation with all its limitations for us. People with MS feel that staff and others can, at the end of the day, go home and enjoy life, whereas they cannot. The person with MS will quite often make sure that he is not forgotten. He will raise his voice; he will make demands; he will complain perhaps and ask to be given attention. Perhaps as a loud cry — 'I'm here, don't forget it!' The tragedy is perhaps at times that staff, family and friends do not take the reasons for patients' anger into account and take their anger as a personal attack when it has originally nothing or little to do with the people who become the target of it. By receiving anger in return for his own, the person with MS has his hostile behaviour further fed. Relatives, family and staff may then use avoidance, shortened visits or shortened ward rounds or make the anger into an unnecessary argument by defending their stand, not knowing that the issue is often totally irrelevant.

People working in MS centres, as well as family members if this anger occurs at home, should be encouraged to listen to people with MS and at times even *accept some irrational act,* knowing that the relief in expressing it will help the person with MS toward better adaptation to his disease. Family here too can be offered advice to allow the person with MS to express his anger without adding guilt feelings to it, by allowing it to destroy the very relationship that he values most.

The most satisfactory or healthy way of dealing with aggressive drives in general, of course, is through the ego-defence mechanism of sublimation by which the aggressive drive is channelled into acceptable pursuits. These pursuits obviously will vary from person to person, but could include discussing politics in a group situation, slinging off anger at politicians perhaps, table sports, space invader games, aggressively belting some clay around in preparation for pot making and talking about their feelings to a non-condemning therapist.

On the other hand, there is a situation in which some people with MS do not express their anger and this too creates a difficult situation.[12] The problem here is that when anger is felt toward a person on whom one is dependent, it is feared that a display of anger might alienate the person who satisfies this dependency need, resulting in ultimate rejection by that person. It is for this reason that anger is then suppressed. Also, the non-affected partner may feel anger toward the MS person, but suppresses it, feeling that expressing anger produces guilt feelings in himself due to the felt unacceptability of expressing anger towards disabled or sick people. Again, in this situation, a psychologist, or others dealing with psychological aspects of the person with MS, can help this person and indeed his family by allowing expression of the anger, looking for the causes of the anger and, through this awareness, can open communication between the two people between whom the anger exists.

MANAGEMENT OF DEPRESSION

Drug therapy generally assumes a major role in the management of people who express depressive syndromes. Research into depression in MS by Whitlock (see Chapter 7) shows that although many people with MS will develop depression as an understandable reaction to their disease, others more clearly suffer from endogenous depression which could be the direct consequence of cerebral damage. Pathological evidence implicates areas of the brain such as the frontal lobe and other parts of the limbic system whose impairment, through disease, often results in serious depression or, less frequently, mania. However, as stated in the beginning, a preparatory depression has often been noticed as a result of fear of impending losses. However, a reactive depression accompanied by unrealistic guilt or shame is also frequently seen.

The initial reaction to depressed people is usually to try to cheer them up, to tell them not to take things so grimly or so hopelessly. This is often, however, an expression of our own needs, our own inability to tolerate a long face over an extended period of time. However, it is often contraindicated to tell people not to be sad, since all of us are tremendously sad or depressed when we experience losses. Here, the support one can give to both the person with MS and family members is to allow the expression of these feelings of sorrow, because all of this will make the final adaptation to the symptoms much easier and both the person with MS and his family will be grateful to those who can sit with them through this stage of depression without constantly telling them not to be sad. In this depression, the person with MS has much to share in fact, and requires many verbal interactions and often active intervention on the part of people from many disciplines. To be allowed to express their grief, their fears and fantasies to someone who can sit quietly and listen, tends to aid tremendously in the total adaptation process. In fact, as it has been once said, to give words to fear can be tremendously alleviating of depressed and anxious feelings.

During the years of contact with persons with MS, it has become apparent that even the most accepting, sometimes called realistic, of people with MS always leave the possibility open for some cure— for the discovery of some new drug or for some other miracle. This hope, it is felt, maintains people with MS through their suffering. It is the feeling that all this must have some meaning, will pay off eventually if they can only endure it for a little while longer. It is also a hope that occasionally sneaks in— as someone expressed it in a group therapy once, 'all this is just a nightmare and not true'— that they will wake up one morning to be told that a new drug has been found which seems promising, that they will use it on him, and that he may be the chosen special person with MS to play a special role in life. It helps people with MS to endure more tests and, in a sense, it is a rationalisation for their suffering at times. Most people with MS show the greatest confidence if staff will allow for such hope. Relatives here can also be of help, but frequently do not know anything about the MS condition or the course it may or may not take. They therefore find it difficult to support the person with MS in this type of hope, and they themselves too might lose hope and, because of this, are unable to support the member of their family with MS. Hope, however, should be offered in spite of bad news.

Another factor that needs to be taken into account in dealing with depression, preparatory depression and anxiety is that the same person may wish to talk about the unpleasant aspects of life one day and the very pleasant ones the next. The staff and family should respect these wishes. Also, as the disease progresses, a person tends to feel the possibilities shrink, expectations and requirements becoming smaller, and may try to deal with life by living for a possible remission whenever it might occur. When such a person feels bad, he wants to be left alone, to withdraw, and attempts to sleep. When he feels better, he will let people know that he is ready to communicate again and become sociable. Insight into this feeling might help the family to deal with the depression and may alleviate anxiety in staff who might feel that this person should talk about his sad feelings.

THE PROBLEM OF CURIOSITY

Adjustment by the family to the demands of MS and its psychosocial consequences requires communication about disability. However, many people with MS reject interest by their family and relatives in these aspects. There are a number of reasons for this. The first reason clearly is that talking about the particular disabling symptoms will reactivate unpleasant feelings in the person with MS. The second reason, which again is frequently brought up at group sessions, is that the person with MS frequently regards his disability as something to be ashamed of; in other words it is a mark of inferiority and therefore should not be discussed because it emphasises his inferior status. However, at the same time, all people with MS want what they actually go through to be understood by the other person. Silence is therefore no solution. For some people disabled with MS, particularly those visibly disabled, it is a social fact anyway and hiding their symptoms is no longer possible. For others, the social strain and superficial personal relations which result from not talking about it are frequently intolerable and cause excess stress and, at times, depression.

The person with MS is thus faced with a conflict produced by:

1. a tendency to shield the self from prying eyes and curious minds for the reasons stated; and
2. the desire to reveal oneself to be understood.

The resolution to this conflict can lie in:

1. provision of more information to family and relatives about the MS condition;
2. making people with MS aware of this conflict;
3. working through the conflict during therapy sessions, which can include group therapy.

THE PROBLEM OF SOCIAL ACCEPTANCE

People disabled with MS who are part of the author's group therapy frequently report that they are being left out of social groups and attribute this to a difference in perception of the limitations that MS imposes on their behaviour. The distinct feeling from the group is that those non-disabled overestimate the limitations of the disease. In fact, talking to many non-disabled, it is clear that they feel that exclusion from group activity is a sensible acceptance of reality and, yet, this is seen by the person with MS as social exclusion.[16]

The support one can give here to a person with MS as well as the non-disabled, including his family, is that advice needs to be given to leave the decision making to the person with MS since he is frequently able to participate in a way compatible with his own interests, but not considered satisfying perhaps for the non-disabled. For example, watching a game instead of playing it might still be acceptable to a person disabled by MS, and he wants to participate on this level as it includes the social interaction that comes with it after the game. One should therefore work out with the MS person what he feels able to do, accepting his fluctuating energies but certainly making him aware to *'state his preference'*.

MISFORTUNE AND DISABILITY

Misfortune and disability involve the loss of something valued. Therefore, the person who experiences misfortune is generally expected to suffer and mourn his loss. This has become very clear in therapy sessions both with people with MS and the families involved. For example, it has become an apparent insistence by some relatives who value their own marriage, that a person whose marriage has been put in serious jeopardy through the course of MS should act like an unfortunate person. As long as people with MS and their relatives and families act in a depressed manner, everything is regarded as all right. However, if people do not act in an unfortunate manner, the non-affected spouse or family members or relatives suspect simulating or see the person with MS as emotionless or having no values. For example, in a number of family set-ups, the therapy carried out by the author to ease the transition from living with a severely disabled spouse to living with the fact that, although still married, it was necessary for that spouse to live in a nursing home set-up, resulted in a fairly smooth transition for the non-affected spouse. However, brothers and sisters of the affected person felt that his spouse, by not becoming depressed, was not acting like an unfortunate person whose husband had just been permanently placed in an MS centre, and therefore suspected her of being emotionless and of having no values. Preventative work by increasing coping mechanisms as such, can then create its own problems.

However, this implies that the non-disabled relatives and spouses, in fact society in general, want people with MS and their relatives to behave in a suffering manner. It is felt that this indicates a lack of insight by family, relatives and society in general as to how to view the losses that people experience. The best support to be given here, perhaps to both the person with MS and his family, and indeed to society, is to begin to view the physical loss a person has experienced as the loss of a possession and not of personal characteristics devaluating the person. In other words, it is a part of the body, a tool, not a personal characteristic. Secondly, it will help the non-affected family members, friends and society as well as the person with MS, to evalute any loss in terms of other characteristics. For example, within the broad context of values, including personality characteristics, friendliness and the ability to be a father, the loss of use of the legs can become less important.

THE PROBLEM OF ACCEPTING AND SUPPORT

Most people with MS will accept help and support when necessary, but there is a discrepancy generally between their definition of necessary and that of their family, or even of those involved in treating them. To people with MS, necessary help means assistance that is essential to the attainment of a goal. To the family and even some staff who deal with people with MS, it frequently means assistance that will expedite matters. Therefore, help given is quite frequently inappropriate. The definition of necessary help for the person with MS has two sources.

Source 1. He will reject inessential but useful help because he wants the security of being able to do things on his own. Also, acceptance of help precludes learning, which is his only way to increase his area of free movement: in other words, to achieve independence. It is clear, therefore, that help is seen, if offered in the previous context, as depriving the self of the possibility of advancing towards an important goal having many values:

a. promotion of self-esteem,
b. insurance against future insecurity,
c. increase in social status,
d. protection against becoming spoiled (babied).

Source 2. This includes the fear that if help is accepted, it leads to the assignment of a role which indicates social inferiority. In other words, it leads to status judgements. Help in this regard is seen as a disparaging situation which means:

a. lack of recognition of ability,
b. the implication of pity,
c. the giver being motivated by a need for self-aggrandisement,
d. calling attention to the MS person and placing him apart from the others.

In fact, this calling attention upon ourselves, this feeling of standing out in the crowd, is a fear that many people with MS discuss in the group therapy sessions. It tends to make them feel as though they belong to a minority group but, even more so, that they belong to a socially inferior minority group, so that help is frequently rejected for this reason.

Therefore, the person with MS has to resolve the conflict between two antagonistic situations, these being:

1. desire to achieve maximum independence whilst being treated as anyone else, and yet
2. requiring help that others do not need.

If the person with MS can reorganise the meaning of help and feel that it is offered, not as to a disabled person, but merely as to one who is having difficulty in a particular situation, he has partly solved the conflict. In other words, disability should be seen by him as not detracting from his personal worth and setting him apart, but merely as causing difficulties in certain performances of behaviour. Such a view, of course, should ideally be held by the family and society in general.

One can further help the person with MS who is facing conflict in this area by making him aware that many acts are performed by the non-disabled to help each other and disabled people without reference to disability, and that neither performance nor omission of help can be taken as a criterion as to how he is regarded as a person.

OTHER FAMILY RELATIONSHIPS

Outside the marital relationship mentioned so far, there are many other relationships within the primary unit, each of which can experience possible changes as a result of MS. Take, for example, the situation where the person with MS is single, had MS diagnosed between the ages of 20 and 25 or older and, as a result of symptoms, moves back in with his parents. Such a situation can result in the parents reassuming their previous parental role with a tendency to be overprotective. Support here is clearly different but, again, involves both parents and the MS person discussing their feelings with each other in an effort to set boundaries acceptable to both.

Another relationship, that of young children with an MS-disabled parent, can be helped by encouraging these children to express their feelings on paper through their drawing of the family. This approach also gives some insight into how these children view their disabled parent. For example, one 8-year-old boy drew his wheelchair-fast father as a person standing with vague feet. Two months later, he drew his father with nothing below the belt. Six months after that, he drew dad in a wheelchair, making roaring engine noises as he did so, proclaiming it to be the sportscar wheelchair.

Older children need different support. Some of these children, for example, appear to shield themselves from stigma by not bringing friends home. Role changes within the family for these children too can produce their own stresses.

It is felt that for both younger and older children, the teachers too should at times be involved, particularly where school performances can be affected due to the MS influence on the family home situation.

COMING TO TERMS WITH MS DISABILITY

This is, of course, the greatest problem for the family and the MS-disabled person alike. In this regard though, it is important to remember that all marital relationships, and indeed all relationships within the primary unit, experience stresses and strains and that they pull at all the family members and stretch the ties that bind, even under ideal conditions. If, however, one adds to this condition the circumstances of MS, particularly in the way it re-defines the lives of those who have it and the lives of those nearest and dearest, the impact can obviously become overwhelming. However, with support, the family and person with MS can develop a number of effective ways of coming to terms with MS. The ineffective ways noticed have included:

1. efforts to equal able-bodied persons;
2. rejection of help;
3. avoidance of discussing disability.

Coming to terms is also made difficult for those with MS due to the already stated contradiction between the use of the word patient and yet not acting within the sick role. In this regard, the word 'accept' is one that presents another conflict. Again, looking at *The Oxford Dictionary*, the word 'accept' is described as meaning 'to allow the truth of'. In the case of MS, of course, this creates tremendous conflict. By allowing the truth of or the fact that he has MS (which, according to both staff and people with MS, really means accepting all the symptoms and reactions that come with the disease), the person with MS is still told to fight it. The conflict here is: say you have it, accept it and yet fight it! The very word 'accept' seems to be in contradistinction to the word 'fight'. Thus a person with MS may be best helped by changing the wording to 'accept the diagnosis' and by accepting perhaps that what we know about MS is still limited, and even that what we know is not necessarily applicable to each individual, and that rather than accepting symptoms, we should look at what each person with MS can do to change them or, perhaps with the help of rehabilitation personnel, to minimise their impact. Psychological and social symptoms are frequently those over which the person can establish some control, particularly with the support of his family, his own insight, the development of new coping strategies and the support of rehabilitation staff. This control is in contrast to the lack of control over the physical progression of the disease. However, this control over the psychological and social aspects of the disease is difficult to achieve on one's own and also for the family in general, and does need enormous support along some of the lines suggested in this chapter and further highlighted and explored in the next chapters.

REFERENCES

1. Barrett F.M. (1981). *Sexuality and Mutliple Sclerosis*. Toronto: Multiple Sclerosis Society of Canada.
2. Hartings M.F., Pavlou M.M., Davis F.A. (1976). Group counselling of MS patients. *Journal of Chronic Diseases*; **29**:65–73.
3. Surridge D. (1969). An investigation into some psychiatric aspects of multiple sclerosis. *British Journal of Psychiatry*; **115**:749–64.
4. Weinstein E.A. (1970). Behavioural aspects of multiple sclerosis. *Modern Treatment*; **7**(5):962–8.
5. Simons A.F. (1981). *Multiple Sclerosis: Family Reaction*. University of Queensland: Ongoing PhD Thesis.
6. Simons A.F. (1981). *Supporting People with MS and their Families*. Paper delivered as an opening address for Patient Services, National Conference on MS, Melbourne.
7. Vowels L. (1978). *Memory Impairment in Multiple Sclerosis*. Paper delivered at National Conference on MS, Sydney.
8. Whitlock F.A., Siskind D.M.M. (1980). Depression as a major symptom of multiple sclerosis. *Journal of Neurology, Neurosurgery and Psychiatry*; **43**:861–5.
9. Kahana, E., Leibowitz U., Alter M. (1971). Cerebral multiple sclerosis. *Neurology (Minneapolis)*; **21**:1179–85.
10. Pulton T.W. (1977), Multiple sclerosis: a social–psychological perspective. *Physical Therapy*; **57**:170–73.
11. Simons A.F. (1980). *Multiple Sclerosis: Perceptions of Health Care and the Quality of Life*. University of Queensland: MSPD Thesis.
12. Simons A.F. (1981). *Society's Reaction to Disability*. IYDP Seminar, Camp Duckadang.
13. National Council for Health Statistics (1970). *Selected Symptoms of Psychological Stress*. New York: National Council for Health Statistics.
14. Tucket D. (1976). *Medical Sociology*. London: Tavistock.
15. Burnfield P. (1978). Sexual problems and multiple sclerosis. *British Journal of Family Planning*; **4**:2–5.
16. Simons A.F. (1981). *Changing Community Attitudes*. Paper delivered at Sporting Wheelies Seminar, Brisbane.

One Man's Experience with Multiple Sclerosis

John Brown, now in his early forties, is a full-time professional journalist in New Zealand and an MS sufferer. In this chapter he gives an account of how MS has affected his life and his efforts to come to terms with its effects. Being closely involved with MS societies in 11 countries and having undertaken several periods of study and overseas travel, he is in a unique position to supply insights into the work of these societies.

Growing up in a small New Zealand city demands conformity. I did not conform. By the time I reached puberty at 13 years of age I was well developed physically but, unlike my sports-crazed male classmates, I was unable to function with their 'macho' abilities. I got too tired and I often stumbled. As a clumsy, rather ungainly teenager I suffered from regular bouts of broken sleep which my parents described as 'growing pains'. These intense bone pains went on unexplained and unexamined by doctors until I was about 16 years old. I continued to be a rather awkward teenager. But at 17, wonder of all wonders, I succeeded in beating all my classmates in regular contests of rope climbing!

Our gymnastics teacher had been a New Zealand Army 'bull' major. He had little tolerance for physical malingerers. I dreaded each enforced exercise as I moved ungainly from one piece of gym equipment to the other. The balancing exercises left me a staggering wreck. Then it happened! Down came the huge ropes one day from the high ceiling of the school gymnasium. A hoist up from the teacher; a few rudimentary instructions and I had reached the roof line way ahead of my more macho mates. I'd had my first individual sporting success. My arms and shoulders became something like a new friend. Praise flooded over me from my gym teacher. I no longer felt a dropout in the sporting arena.

New self-confidence took the place of seeing myself as a failure. I started to excel at short-distance running. My bicycle became a good training agent. However, despite enormous encouragement and personal determination, I never became anything like proficient at that most Kiwi of sports— rugby. In the mid-1950s, not being a rugby player was a sure way to become a social dropout amongst one's peer group. I felt isolated and began to devote more time to academic work than sport. My chosen friends too were academics, not sports fanatics. I did well at school studies and entered university and later teachers' training college. By the time I reached 18, I knew that nothing short of a miracle would give me the physical ability of my fellows. I had the same equipment as them, I looked the same, but real physical achievement eluded me.

By the time I had completed three years at university, I had found satisfying compensations in student life for my utter failure to conform to the small-town New Zealand syndrome and its fanaticism in sport. Then, however, the spectre of the 'physical' intruded again. As a teacher trainee, it was mandatory to be able to swim. Each time my fellow trainees romped about the pool, I clung to the side, fearful of venturing too far out. I was taught over a period of two years to enjoy the physical sensation of relaxation in water. I even managed to move out into the 'deep' part, but I never became a swimmer. Fortunately the regulations were waived for me. What is more, I did become a competent swimming teacher as part of my general teaching.

At age 21, I took up my first full-time teaching post and my arch enemy rugby reared its ugly head again! Horror of horrors, I was expected to coach the infernal game, which I did reluctantly. Then I suddenly discovered my true sport— soccer. I had never played the game before and could no more manipulate my clumsy legs to cope with the demands of this game than for the Kiwi 'religion' of rugby. However, I was the teacher and I did become, after careful study and encouragement from a small group of Dutch parents, a regional representative soccer coach for junior players. Somewhere in the back of my mind I then remembered the rope-climbing experience!

Soccer gave me an important involvement in sport. I was almost a real Kiwi through this sport! By the time I had reached 24 years of age, my eyes were beginning to show signs of deterioration. Always short sighted, I had worn glasses since my mid-teens. I rode a motor cycle. I danced, but always with sympathetic and skilled partners. I continued to play the piano, which had been a long-term hobby and which compensated somewhat for my lack of sporting ability. Life seemed fine. I became engaged to marry. My teaching career was satisfying and successful. However, a routine visit to a doctor soon changed all that!

Doing part-time university studies, I was expected to have a medical check each year with the student health service. I was seated when a young doctor came into the room. He did his routine tests. As I left the room he said: 'Do you always walk like that?' 'I've always been a bit clumsy and stumble a lot', I replied. What followed changed my life!

I was given what I now know only too well to be the standard set of preliminary neurological tests for multiple sclerosis. In quick succession, I went to a neurologist and was examined and admitted to hospital for a battery of tests. After these tests, which included the inevitable lumbar puncture and myelogram, my wife and I were left to reflect in ignorance on this unexpected sudden medical intrusion into our lives.

A week after leaving hospital, I was told that I had a suspected tumour on my spine . . . but no answer was given as to why I walked differently and why I was having frequent 'dizzy' spells. The news of the non-diagnosis contributed further complications to a marriage which was already failing for other reasons. The word 'tumour' knocked my wife. Emotionally, I let things flow over me. My marriage finally broke up. The doctors' failure to explain the symptoms sparked off the final messy break-up.

I left teaching and took up a less physically strenuous job as a journalist. After a year, I returned to my old university city to work for a newspaper there. I felt at home amongst its scholastic towers. My walking became more awkward; my eyes began to 'jump'; the dizzy spells increased in intensity. After referral to a university-based neurologist, I went back into hospital for another round of tests and my new specialist consulted with my original neurologist. At last I was given the diagnosis: multiple sclerosis! This was almost five years after that fateful visit to the student health service.

On a cold dismal winter's day in Dunedin, I visited the neurologist to hear the results of my tests and two weeks in hospital. With refreshing candour, MS was explained to me. However, still I was bewildered; things still did not make much sense.

'You'll have to take life easy. Things will change. You may have to give up work,' the doctor said. 'To hell I will' I thought.

And then the worst part came. I had to leave that silent building on my own and stagger up a crowded street filled with Friday night shoppers. I gazed in vain through a mist of disbelief for someone to share my awful truth with. I felt lost; utterly alone!

An unsuspecting professional contact tapped me out of my dreamy path: 'Hi John . . . what's up?'. My flood of words in response almost knocked the poor man, who was a recent Dutch settler. He listened sympathetically but had to go home, despite my need for company. I continued to wander that night. I had no car. I was too tired, too dispirited to try to find others to tell my fears to. Joining my workmates for the normal Friday night 'session' in the local pub was an easy way out! Although I intended not to tell any of them, I still did, leaving them as bewildered as I felt.

That weekend, I visited many friends looking for some reassurance:

some knowledge, some hope! What I did not realise then, was that all the help I needed was around me in my workmates and friends. First though, I had to come to terms with this, now labelled, condition. How could I though, when I could hardly even pronounce it properly.

I became a dreary soul at that time. I worked like a slave. My fellow journalists left me to it. I won a couple of journalism prizes. Work became my loving partner; my workmates my supporters.

When I left that newspaper two years later, I learnt that two of my junior colleagues had taken the trouble to find out something about MS. They had gone to talk to my editor and had offered, after I was diagnosed, to do my typing for me as they thought I might not be able to do it myself. Yes! work was my supporter all right!

An even harder step in the period of diagnosis was telling my parents. Neither understood. How could they anyway — particularly as even I knew precious little. They did want to help though and bought me a badly needed car.

What I wanted even more though was a shoulder to cry on. This I finally found in the understanding wife of a life-long friend. The 'spell' was broken and by the time I was promoted to a job on my country's second largest morning newspaper, I thought I could forget about that uncomfortable diagnosis. But I did not know MS and I reckoned without its deceitful habit of coming back and hitting you with full fury!

Sharing a flat with some colleagues, I led a full social life. I even took steps to find out what the local Multiple Sclerosis Society was doing. My first visit there shocked me. The sight of all those people in wheelchairs made my blood run cold. I wasn't like them — how little I knew!

During Christmas 1972, one of my flatmates returned from work to find me almost in tears. The sight in my right eye had gone and I was terrified. He postponed his holiday until I had visited a doctor. I was not too sure of the quality of medical advice I might get though. My worst fears were well founded when the GP told me to take some Valium and rest up. I waited, and so did my friend. A week later, my eyesight returned to normal. Still no one told me why this could happen. For an answer to that, I had to wait a further six months when I returned to hospital for a reassessment, this time at my own request. The doctor had told me to come back if I wanted further help. I sure did. MS was beginning to get in the way of my life. It was only by chance that I did find out on that visit what had happened to my eyesight, as my neurologist explained the temporary blindness to a group of medical students within my hearing. Remaining politely silent as I lay on an examination couch at the front of that crowded lecture theatre, I thought: 'Bloody doctors!'

The doctor went on to explain to the students that my temporary blindness confirmed the diagnosis of MS, making me think of the huge gaps in information with which most people with MS have to live. Questions started flooding into my mind as I lay there. Perhaps the fact that I was having difficulty in maintaining a normal sex life had something to do with MS? However, this was not the place to sit up and ask questions of this specialist. The devil in me, however, gave me a great urge to ask the doctor, in front of his willing students, a few pointed questions. They would have been shocked I'm sure if I— the patient— had dared to ask to be consulted, to be involved!

As the students did their neurological 'prodding', as they gazed into my eyes with their ophthalmoscopes for the tell-tale signs of optic neuritis, I started to think that those of us with MS held the trump card. It just might be that we knew something more than the medicos did. Sure, the condition was confusing, but we were living— and loving— with it. It seemed to me there and then, that it was high time changes were made and that the voice of people with MS should begin to feature in the history of the condition in New Zealand and perhaps other countries.

Little did I realise then what 'rebellious' thoughts those were, particularly for my country in the early 1970s. However, having those thoughts and acting on them was the second big change that MS made in my life.

I returned to work full of determination to get something positive going for people with MS and, in the process, find out answers to some pretty fundamental questions myself.

A young man of 22 made the matter more urgent. He came to me through a mutual friend, asking for help. He said he knew another 'friend' who was about to marry but also had MS and was having problems maintaining a normal sex life. This all sounded very familiar to me. It wasn't long before the young man admitted that it was he who had MS and could I help?

Precious little written information was available in New Zealand at that time for people with MS. No one bothered to ask us what we wanted to know.

We became an angry pair of MS people who went to visit a sympathetic Danish-trained doctor one day to badger him with important questions about MS. We left the surgery firmly convinced that information was available and that it was up to us to help break down community suspicion and ignorance and patients' doubts about MS. We started.

The young man got married and now leads a happy life overseas. For my part, I've tried to act, largely because of my profession, as an unofficial 'stirrer' on behalf of MS people. This has not always made me popular with others.

Carried on a wave of enthusiasm, I accepted nomination as the first person with MS to stand for the executive of the local MS society. I was elected, but told soon afterwards by a former part-time worker for that MS society that I should not be on the board as I had MS. 'How bloody stupid,' I thought, marking in my mind that that critic certainly did not deserve a place on the board ever. Fortunately she left the society altogether and gradually there started a process of change within the society. However, a change also started in me; one which I was totally unprepared to face: depression!

When this hit me, I tried to fight. I struggled to work on my walking sticks each day. I even thought of suicide. I thought how much easier it would be to become 'disabled', to be listed as one of the nation's statistics and simply give up. Living alone did not help, but my understanding doctor did. He was the same Danish GP who had helped before and he spent many hours in personal counselling. Through him, I learnt that depression cannot be 'fought'. The harder we try to do this, the deeper we tend to become involved in its sticky clutches. Helped by drug therapy, I came through this first totally debilitating bout of departure from real life. I even wrote about it. Somehow I'd looked fear in the face and managed to meet its persistent stare. But, as my doctor warned, depression came back.

This most unwelcome of MS symptoms has been with me for most years. I've even been a full-time patient in a psychiatric hospital for a short time because of it. I have learned to see depression without fear, to accept help and to grow through it. My time in hospital also taught me a lot more about human relationships, about myself and about the natural anger that is part of a disabled person's efforts to cope with life. I found a new energy in my dreaded brush with depression. But I did not attempt to do it on my own. In coping with my depressed feelings, I found a new closeness with my workmates. It was vital to me to share as much with people around me and I found that they too had their fears.

Awarded, in 1976, a New Zealand Government Winston Churchill Travelling Study Award, I was given a unique opportunity to travel overseas and see what other countries were doing for people with MS. I visited Holland, Denmark, West Germany, Belgium, England, parts of the USA and Canada. I also became a delegate to the Thirtieth Conference of The National MS Society of the USA and attended the World MS Conference in Toronto. I visited clinics and MS agencies. I learnt a great deal and, in the process, overdid my activity in every way— physically, socially and psychologically. But I did it and grew through it.

A professional windfall enabled me to make another trip in 1977 to Holland for the World MS Conference and also for a holiday with friends in Denmark, Germany and England. Hard saving gave me another opportunity for overseas travel in 1979. This took me to Vienna for that year's world MS Conference and also to Denmark, Germany, Switzerland and Zimbabwe, where I visited MS contacts. On my way home, I stopped off in Australia to attend the Third National MS Conference there. By then, I was awash with MS information and ideas!

My constant and very necessary companion on all these long journeys was my wheelchair. I had fought against the idea of using one until a Dutch physiotherapist told me that it was simpler for me, and indeed others like me, to make temporary use of this aid, so as not to over-tire myself. This was another breakthrough that required, and still requires, reasonable explanation to others. It is far easier to use the chair, and later get up and walk about with the energy thus saved, than to struggle about on sticks all the time.

On my first visit to Holland, it was pointed out to me that people with MS were 'people first and patients second'. This phrase became a beacon to me when I gave a series of public lectures on MS throughout my own country in 1977. In all, I spoke to 30 different groups that year. My 1976 trip had taught me a new skill— public speaking! I had one big advantage — I was beginning to know my topic well: 'MS and how to live with it'.

However, my views did not always meet with the acclaim of others. New Zealand is not seen by me as a country where new views are readily accepted. It was hard work to promote my view that disabled people are very much part of the community. Overseas experience, however, had taught me that and my profession fortunately made it possible to promulgate that view. I was variously labelled as 'dangerous', 'an activist', 'a red' and 'a stirrer'. The Establishment of the Disabled Persons' Movement in New Zealand was not used to having their bricks and mortar institutional philosophy for the disabled questioned. It must have been hard for the Establishment when they were faced with a disabled journalist who had learnt most of his tricks from examples seen in Denmark, Sweden, Holland and Britain. In those countries, shutting people away from the mainstream of society is not accepted as 'normal'.

The Vice-President of New Zealand's MS National Society warned that 'talking about the success of the Danish MS Society had no relevance to New Zealand as Denmark was a socialist country'! Those types of comments I was forced to counter. However, the view around in New Zealand is that we somehow are far ahead of the rest of the world in MS care. This I know to be plainly inaccurate. Why even now, in 1983, we still have not even got a professionally organised national MS office; there are still no full-time national officers. However, I do know that change is afoot.

In the frenetic activity with which I became involved to help reform the local MS society, I soon learnt that not all people were averse to change. The many thousands of dollars spent by the Government and myself on overseas trips have not gone to waste. My fellow 200 people with MS in Christchurch wanted to make use of what I had learnt and went about it in a progressive and carefully planned manner.

As an agent of change, I had a unique responsibility to those less fortunate MS sufferers. Yes, I'm not afraid to use the word 'sufferer' from time to time, for we all do suffer and we would be naive in the extreme if we did not admit it.

I believe that in the best of all possible worlds, we have a joint responsibility to make MS organisations around the world more in tune with what we have to live with. Some organisations achieve this result in a positive manner. Others, however, seem more interested in ego trips for their professional officers than in consultation with their clients — the people with MS and those who support them.

In my home city, the local MS society has become a trail blazer. It does consult, and acts on the results. We now have the country's only full-time professional director working alongside those with MS and their helpers. Slowly, New Zealand is developing a system which ensures that information takes the place of the fear, frustration and ignorance that surround MS.

When I visited him in Gottingen in 1976, the German 'master' of MS research— Professor Bauer— told me in his calm manner that 'activitiy is your great ally . . . inactivity your natural enemy'. For example, I learned that activity is vital. It does not have to be physical. We have got to learn new ways to use our bodies, our minds and our emotions. As we live with MS, subtle changes occur in our personality. Perhaps we get angry more often or cry a little more. We have got to share such things. For me, it's been a matter of realising that the most vital thing is friendship; but this requires special efforts on the part of the MS sufferer. If we as disabled people want integration, then we have a responsibility to fight for that right. It's not always easy. Sure, when you are first diagnosed, there are friends everywhere wanting to help. Time dulls these contacts and some will drift away. Those who stay and the new friends you make will support you if they are given the chance to know your needs — if they see you are doing your bit too.

When the subtle cloud of tiredness and lethargy creeps over us, it seems so much easier to curl up like a well-fed cat and let life flow over us. That is exactly what it will do if that is your reaction.

It is often a matter of picking our task, examining the possibilities and priorities; then get stuck into it. Other people will help, but the initiative must come from us. Okay, you might get fed up with other people telling you to 'fight', but if we don't, then there is precious little point in being here anyway. This is where we, as MS sufferers, have a very special part to play in our own battle to live with MS.

The front line for this battle must be our own MS organisation. It is not much use sitting back and saying that the MS society 'does not do much'. The question we must ask ourselves is, 'What can I do for it?' If it is not providing the service that you think it should, then you are probably not the only one who thinks that way. MS societies are there for people with MS. They are not there to provide an easy professional road for non-MS people.

Every one of the 2 million people with MS around the world, their families and their supporters, have a common need — to make the best possible use of the lives of MS sufferers. There is no way this can be done alone. We have got to reach out. Learning to know how and when to do that is our ball game. It certainly will mean change. Just as certainly, it will mean new horizons, new challenges, new friends, and new hope!

One Woman's Experience with Multiple Sclerosis

Florence Lowry was diagnosed as suffering from MS a week before her marriage at the age of 20. Now, some 20 years later, she describes the effects it has had on her life and the ways in which she has learnt to cope with it. After a lapse of some years, during which time she brought up a family, Florence has returned to professional singing and in this chapter relates the long climb back to the active life she now leads.

I am tired. After 20 years of living with multiple sclerosis, it's the exhaustion that is toughest to endure. Before being diagnosed at 20, the eye trouble and the bladder infections were irritants, brushed aside in an active life: singing, theatre, teaching and a man, who did not ask, but told me I was going to marry him. And then you find out 'it's multiple sclerosis' a week before the wedding.

Try learning about multiple sclerosis on a honeymoon! You learn together and you wonder who is being hurt the most. Spend close to half of the first six years of your marriage in hospitals with only the strength to lie there and cry for yourself, unable to cope with the strangled look of helplessness of your partner.

But you learn. You fight off the depression and adjust to a life not of your choosing but of what has been dealt. The disease teaches you that to ignore it or to rebel will only lead to exacerbation. Your family (now including two children) tries to accept and understand. You add the pluses and appreciate the remissions and find, if you are lucky, you can cheat this strange condition in your central nervous system.

I have gone back to my singing. I have had to pace myself. It could not be done overnight. My first supper club date was over New Year. A full house was listening to me and nobody in that audience could see that I had multiple sclerosis. I was tired by the third set but the applause was worth it. I have not beaten mutliple sclerosis but I have leared to live around it.

Painful memories mingle with the joy of youth. I had been accepted into the radio–television arts course at a prominent college. I never could understand the intricacies of the control room or a television camera but being on stage, on camera and popular were exhilarating enough. The ophthalmologist thought the jittery optic nerve was just from overdoing. 'Maybe he's right, I sure am tired but there's a fraternity party tonight I would hate to miss.' I was there.

'Darn bladder! Another infection? Since finishing school, it has been work through the day to pay the rent and the theatre group in the evenings, always the chance for a break as a budding actress or singer and the weekend classes to teach theatre arts to children are fun! Peter is picking me up after the third act but no cast party tonight, I just want to go cuddle up in his arms and maybe I won't feel so tired.'

It was my family doctor who gently but firmly insisted on my going into hospital for neurological tests. I had seen the neurologist she sent me to, but now they wanted to do more than tickle me with pins. She knew I was getting married soon.

Each test was worse than the others, but the uncertainty was the worst part. I had a headache from a lumbar puncture when Peter visited me one afternoon. Maybe that is why I failed to notice how concerned he was about me or to ask why he had been delayed in the hall talking to the neurologist. He soon had me laughing but all I really wanted was some rest.

He had a hard time getting me to laugh in those years when I was learning the reality of multiple sclerosis. Tensions and jitters were bad enough at my parents' home the weekend before the wedding. My doctor could not face me. She told me over the telephone. Peter and my father were chatting in the living room. My mother was starting to prepare dinner. My world went black: 'Florence, the tests show that you have multiple sclerosis.'

Maybe the worst trauma was the truth. By my wedding day, I was limping; my entire left side was numb; both eyes were suffering from inflamed optic nerves: the wedding was a blur. When people ask me about my wedding, all I can mention is the unseasonable heat— it was 95°F— and the surprise when my new husband answered the toast to the bride with a speech that had the overheated families and friends laughing themselves off the hard church-hall chairs.

What new bride takes medical books and Multiple Sclerosis Society literature on her honeymoon? We read them together. We phoned from a resort to ask my doctor what to do about a worsening bladder infection and she laughed it off as the 'honeymoon syndrome'. We knew it was not that.

The medical books and literature were no help. We found it impossible to understand my personal needs and condition from the vague literature of the Society (which seemed more interested in raising funds than me) and the skimpy mumbo-jumbo of the medical texts. The future did not exist; I lived each day.

Friends were the major problem. I hated the solicitous patronising. I resented those who made light of it. 'What now?' or 'What next?' led the cacophony of growing concerns. I would abuse my husband when he was overly concerned about me. He became an object upon which I could vent my frustrations— one moment with anger and the next with sexual demands. My life became over-dramatised as I became the actress caught up in a crazy over-indulgence in the Stanislavsky method: I wanted to go back to being me but the disease had become my only role.

I would damn the rain when it reminded me with hypersensitivity of my health. Depression led quickly to despair and thoughts of self-destruction. I would find myself looking for scapegoats as a way of surviving.

All the doctors could do was treat the symptoms. Steroids— cortisone and ATCH — took their toll: three unsuccessful pregnancies, against doctors' orders, told me the facts and depression became ever more acute.

The acting and teaching children were set aside in favour of my husband: I told myself. After the second bout of six weeks in hospital, it also meant an end to any value of myself as being able to hold a job or earn a living. My husband was coming home from work to look after me; suffering the abuse, frustration and lack of control of my emotional states.

I could not face seeing another patient. My Aunt Grace— not a blood relation— had multiple sclerosis. I was hardly like her. I did not want to be. Before, I had always felt sorry for her: she had been in a wheelchair for years. I hated it in the hospital when they would put me in a wheelchair. I would have preferred to crawl on the floor.

What was most frightening in those early years was the lack of any certainty to my life. The kindest comment the doctors could make was that they could not even guess what the future held for me.

But, I was lucky. Oh, how lucky! Even with those repeated, long-lasting exacerbations of those early years, followed by weeks and months of physiotheraphy, I never suffered any permanent physical disability. I remember a few years ago, standing talking to a young person with multiple sclerosis who was in a wheelchair, and she looked up at me and said, 'I like you. But I hate you. Damn you for having multiple sclerosis and not being like me!'. I understood.

It would be great to say that one day I learned how to cope with multiple sclerosis. The frustrations are always with me. What I have learned is how to cope with myself. Nobody could help me. Yes, some people along the way have pointed me in the right direction. I have learned from other patients, through my efforts to help them; I have learned much from what is now being written about this disease; but mainly I have learned from those who love me to place a value on being me.

It has taken years of ups and downs. I once spent six weeks in the psychiatric ward of my local hospital because the stress and depression had gone beyond my or my family's ability to handle it. It was the realisation, once I started to listen, that much of the problem was related to my physical health at the time. I was far more confident leaving than when I signed myself in.

At one time, hospitals had become a haven. Frequent exacerbations had meant many months in the cocoon of others worrying for me. I was willing to resort to self-pity and let others do the positive things for me. Even at home, it was easier to let my family look after me than to come to grips with what I should expect of myself.

It is much easier to blame others than yourself. 'Let them understand my problem,' you say. You find that friendships cool if you spend your time with friends telling them your problems. Maybe you should be in a wheelchair so that they could pour out the pity, without you having to try to convince them you need it.

It's a myriad of things that bring you to reality. It's the adorable puppy that your husband places on your bed after another bout in the hospital. It's working to convince the child welfare people that you really should be allowed to adopt a child.

Breaking the barriers of bureaucracy was a challenge; but we convinced them to let us adopt not just one but later another child. It is when your son is 4 years old and is diagnosed as being diabetic that the realisation really hits that you never asked: 'Why me?'

Maybe the realisation comes when a 5 year old has been lifted up to the kitchen counter for his daily injection and complains that it's not fair. Preoccupied with preparing the mix of insulin, you answer, 'Who promised you life would be fair?' Why should we complain about what life has dealt us when it is how we handle it that is really most important?

It would probably surprise many of our friends in our Multiple Sclerosis Society to know that I never really wanted my husband to become as active in it as he did. When he became National President of the Society, I spent many hours at home wishing he would look after the patient there, instead of the tens of thousands across the country.

Not that I have not appreciated the many improvements in the Society over the years. When I first asked my neurologist about the Society, she brushed the question aside with a brusque, 'You don't need them'. Maybe it was the implied 'not yet' that really frightened me. To be fair, it was a small dedicated group of people in the Society in those days, but they had few resources and had to concentrate much of their efforts on fund raising and some very limited services to the most debilitated patients.

In the film *Some Other Time* that my husband produced for the Society, I recognised much of myself in the characters of the two young patients depicted on the screen. It was when I saw how people reacted, though, that I realised that it was an experience that I had shared with many others. I can only hope the film has helped the others who see it as much as it helped me.

All right, 20 years later, I accept it. I have multiple sclerosis. I am not in a wheelchair or even seriously disabled. I am lucky. I am probably among the 48% of patients who will never show any outward signs of the disease. It is still debilitating. I have to bank my energies and use them as effectively as possible. I constantly reorganise my priorities and make sure I am using the energy I have in ways that are important to me and to my family.

Symptoms come and go; but it has been several years now since I have had a serious exacerbation. I live in a northern climate and I hate the winters. Dampness leaves me hypersensitive and depressed; I live with it. My children know that their mother has to have more sleep than most people and she cannot be running up and down stairs all the time to look after their needs and wants.

Sure, I hate the fact that my husband travels so much in his work. I even resent the time he puts into the International Federation of Multiple Sclerosis Societies when he has to travel to what must be exciting parts of the world on its business; but I know what has been achieved there and I can see its worth. I know he has to make a better than average living to pay the extra costs of my having multiple sclerosis; and when you are unable to help defray them, it is difficult to accept.

Even when I went back to singing, he was the one who insisted I do it. We both knew that it would take a lot of work for me to bring my singing skills back to where they were years ago. Surprisingly, they turned out to be better. My vocal coach, who knew me back in the days when I was just one of the many aspirants on some of the young talent showcases on television, said that the maturity had certainly made a difference. Maybe it is more than maturity. Maybe I have learned to live.

My children have noticed a difference. They much prefer to have their mother singing around the house instead of being 'not well' in bed for days on end. When I had the opportunity to appear for a week at one of the popular supper clubs, I could have given a hundred reasons for not doing it. It was my family that convinced me. My husband had the time off and he arranged daily outings for the children and himself so that I could get the extra rest I needed. Yet, he would be waiting up each night when I got home so that I could go over the good and bad points of the evening's performance. I wished he was there every night at the club for the moral support he so generously gives. He is always telling me I can do something when I have doubts. He came down with friends for the next-to-final night and the pride in his face made it all worthwhile.

I'm going to be doing more singing now. No big hits for me though. No circuits, no long club dates. Cutting an album is only a remote possibility. For I have found what I want. I can now live with multiple sclerosis without it beating me. I can live around it by recognising all the good things that life has brought me.

The other day, I was working on a popular song with my vocal coach and when I was finished he gave a low whistle and said, 'Boy, that's sexy!' I laughed and told him it was the words. He said no, it was something I was adding to the number. He is usually right, but all I could think of was that I was feeling good and enjoying life. He told me, whatever it was, to keep it up. I will.

Communicating the Diagnosis

Dr Alexander Burnfield qualified in medicine at the London Hospital Medical College in 1968, and now works as Associate Psychiatrist at the Child and Family Guidance Centre, Winchester, England.

Having had MS for almost 20 years, Dr Burnfield is closely involved with the Crack MS Advisory Committee of the MS Society of Great Britain and Northern Ireland. He lives on a farm with his wife and two foster daughters and, with his wife (also a doctor) provides local counselling for MS sufferers and their relatives.

In this chapter he considers the importance of counselling skills on behalf of doctors and others concerned at the time of diagnosis of MS, and the problems likely to be met with at such a time.

Multiple sclerosis can be difficult to diagnose, yet sufferers must know what is wrong before they can come to terms with the disease. They, and their relatives, need to work through painful feelings before reaching a realistic acceptance of the MS sufferer's limitations and abilities. Honesty and sensitivity are expected, but some doctors lack the counselling skills necessary to communicate the diagnosis properly. Many health professionals and volunteers can help by providing emotional support at the time of diagnosis.

The diagnosis of MS is difficult to make as it depends on a pattern of symptoms and signs occurring over a period of time. There is still no reliable diagnostic test for MS and the disease is often suspected well before it can be confirmed by subsequent events. Yet, an early diagnosis is necessary to exclude treatable conditions (such as spinal tumours) and to meet the needs of research into the disease. Equally important are the emotional needs of the person with MS and his family, who are faced with a frightening experience to which they must adjust before they can plan for the future. Honesty by the doctor will enhance the doctor–patient relationship and will eventually lead to the patient having greater trust in the doctor.

THE PATIENT

A great deal of controversy surrounds the issue of 'telling the patient', and many sufferers claim that they were not told the truth in a straightforward manner.[1,2] Some find out by accident, whilst others have to resort to subterfuge such as steaming open doctors' letters or reading hospital notes upside down. Occasionally the patient's relatives may be informed of the diagnosis, but instructed not to tell the sufferer. This inevitably places a great strain on family relationships.

Even when the diagnosis is certain, a doctor's reluctance to tell may be justified on the grounds that the patient cannot cope with the diagnosis. Yet time after time, MS sufferers speak of relief at knowing their diagnosis. Naturally, many are shocked and distressed, but at least they know the truth and can begin to come to terms with it. The truth is rarely worse than the unknown.

Once the diagnosis of MS is known, a period of adjustment will follow. In many ways, this process parallels that of bereavement. The sufferer has to mourn his lost health and adjust to a 'new identity' — a different picture of himself and his future. He will feel shocked, angry and depressed and may try to deny what has happened to him. This is a normal reaction and it should neither be discouraged nor over-indulged. Counselling at this time may help a sufferer to work through his confused and painful feelings and to accept his limitations.

A particularly distressing feature of MS is the fact that the course of the disease varies greatly from patient to patient. Someone in the early stages lives with an alarming uncertainty about his future. Added to this is the remarkable variability of symptoms within the individual. Not only does the sufferer have to cope with major relapses and remissions but he must also learn to live with ups and downs from day to day and even from hour to hour.

Many MS symptoms are subjective and invisible to other people. Fatigue is a special problem in MS and is made worse by exertion and hot weather. It may fluctuate markedly and can cause a great deal of misunderstanding. This symptom can be extremely disabling for the MS sufferer, but it seems to be less appreciated as a problem by others.

The way in which a person reacts to MS does not necessarily relate to the severity of the disease. A person who is only mildly affected can be psychologically devastated, whilst someone who is severely handicapped might cope well. Many factors play a part in determining an individual's response. These include the effect of the disability on the sufferer's way of life, his personality and the amount of support that he receives from others. A person who is mainly interested in reading might respond better to loss of mobility than to visual impairment, for example.[3]

Adjustment can sometimes be more difficult when symptoms are mild; the sufferer is unsure whether to perceive himself as normal or disabled. When physical signs are more obvious, it may be easier to accept a new identity, but he then has to cope with the stigma of disability. He may try to deny that he is disabled. Some people refuse to use a stick, preferring to stagger about dangerously; neighbours may suspect them of being intoxicated. Others will not adjust their lifestyle and may attempt impossible tasks to prove to themselves that they are still 'normal'. At the other extreme are those people who take to a wheelchair, although they can still walk. In such cases there is often a colluding relative looking for someone to 'mother'. Over-protection may lead to a 'hostile/dependent' relationship in which anger and guilt are mingled.

The person with MS has to find a happy medium between denial on the one hand and giving-in on the other. Only by doing this will he discover his strengths. The best encouragement for a MS sufferer is to be valued and wanted by others. He needs to contribute to society in some way, however small.

THE DOCTOR

Modern physicians are often trained to cure rather than to care for their patients. It seems that medical students are selected primarily for their ability to pass examinations rather than for their more human qualities. Medical training perpetuates this bias, and doctors may come to see their role as that of a technical expert in the diagnosis and treatment of disease. They may prefer to see quick and positive results and may only feel that they have succeeded as doctors if the patient gets better. While being useful in some well-defined medical conditions, this approach can leave the doctor feeling less confident when faced with the vague, often psychosomatic symptoms that he meets in general practice and, more particularly, he may find it difficult to cope with the emotional side of disease.

Technical skills and medical knowledge are not enough. A doctor must combine these with communication and counselling skills if he is to be effective. A balance between bedside manner and technical competence is needed today just as it was at the end of the 16th century when Francis Bacon wrote: 'Physicians are some of them so pleasing and comfortable to the humour of the patient, as they press not the true cure of the disease; and some others are so regular in proceeding according to art for the disease as they respect not sufficiently the condition of the patient. Take one of a middle temper . . .'.[4]

The doctor must also be able to cope with his own feelings of inadequacy or frustration when faced with a MS sufferer, and must not take personally the anger and bitterness projected on to him by his patient. Most importantly, he should realise that he can help his patient best by giving him time and interest and by 'just listening' on occasions. A patient can gain a great deal of relief from sharing his fears and confused feelings and by being accepted as a fellow human being.

A person once diagnosed as having MS must live with a disease which can be both humiliating and depressing. He has to cope with the loss of his health and security as well as changed roles in the family and at work, both so devastating to his self-respect. He can feel angry and may look for someone to blame. He is often eager to find an explanation for his predicament and will easily turn to 'quack' remedies or diets. In both of these circumstances, his doctor will be the natural scapegoat and may be rejected or treated unfairly.

As well as coming to terms with his loss emotionally, the MS sufferer has to cope with the vague initial symptoms of the disease, which are subjective but very real. These symptoms are often difficult to describe without appearing to be 'neurotic' or a 'hypochondriac'. Such labels are sometimes used by doctors but they serve only to undermine the trust and goodwill in the relationship between patient and doctor. Visual or sensory symptoms, and in particular MS fatigue, are hard for sufferers and close relatives to understand. The author has reported his own personal experience of this.[5] It is important that doctors give reassurance and explanation, in order to justify the sick role taken by the sufferer. Because of the difficulties involved in communicating vague symptoms, the sufferer may deny or hide them. Others will exaggerate the symptoms, often in an emotional way, and so perpetuate the doctor's suspicion that they are purely psychological. Both of these strategies inevitably lead to a further breakdown in communication.

THE TIME OF DIAGNOSIS

This is a critical time for all members of the family and it is important that the sufferer and close relatives receive counselling and support as well as accurate information. This, perhaps above all, is the occasion on which the doctor's clinical skills are being tested to the limit. It may be difficult for the doctor to be completely honest at this time for practical reasons. MS is not an easy disease to diagnose and the clinician needs to be sure before communicating a definite opinion. On the other hand, doctors are often discouraged from being open with the sufferer for fear that he or she will not be able to cope emotionally. Yet, knowing the diagnosis may be a relief to the sufferer who is freed from some uncertainty about his fate, and who can then start coming to terms with his condition. Far too often it is the doctor's own feelings that get in the way and he may project his own fears and emotional insecurity on to his patient if he is not sufficiently self-aware.

THE COMMUNICATION

The communication of a disturbing diagnosis or prognosis is not just a question of the transfer of information, but of establishing an appropriate relationship. It is difficult to take in more than a little information in the clinical atmosphere of a consulting room at a time of emotional shock. Patients often forget what they have been told under these conditions and may sometimes deny that they have been given a diagnosis at all.

Diagnosing MS is not just about informing the patient of the facts, but about being sensitive to his emotional needs and reacting appropriately to them. It is often best for a patient and close relative to be seen together for as long as they need to ask questions and to express their feelings. Opportunities must be provided for them to return for more information and support as they require them, and time is necessary for people to work through their feelings of shock, fear, anger and sadness. Some people need to deny part of the truth until they can cope with it all, and skill is needed to assess how much someone really wants to know at any one time. The truth should not be forced down people's throats any more than it should be withheld completely.

When one member of a family is diagnosed as having MS, the whole family will be affected. Children can be very sensitive to anxiety and may become disruptive and attention seeking if their needs are ignored. Facts should be explained to them and, if they are involved in major family decisions, they will not feel excluded and resentful.

The process of grieving that surrounds loss of health and of future security may last a long time. Patients and relatives will need to be given permission to express their natural feelings and this can be painful for those working or living with them. If this process is blocked, then there is a risk that personal and relationship difficulties can occur requiring psychological help at a later stage.

'Telling' the patient and relatives is basically a counselling exercise requiring awareness of psychological processes, self-awareness and relationship skills. But the doctor does not always have sufficient time or even the required counselling skills. Often a nurse, social worker or a psychologist will be able to help on these occasions and may be in a better position to provide the regular in-depth follow-up that is so necessary when a diagnosis of MS has been made. For this to work properly, there must be a shared understanding of each other's roles by medical and non-medical personnel, as well as mutual trust and respect.

Many MS sufferers and their relatives find it helpful to meet others who have successfully come to terms with similar experiences. Self-help groups have grown in the last 20 years and there is undoubtedly a potential for involving other MS sufferers and volunteers in the provision of emotional support. The group counselling of MS patients in a hospital setting has been described;[6] and 'crack MS' self-help groups in the UK now form an important part of the MS society's work in the community.

In the end, there can be no one rule on how to communicate a diagnosis of MS that will suit every occasion, and each doctor and patient has his own views on what is best. Each doctor–patient relationship is unique, and successful communication will largely depend on the sensitivity and clinical judgement of the doctor. For it is the doctor who is ultimately responsible for being receptive to his patient's emotional needs.

REFERENCES

1. Cunningham D. (1977). *Stigma and Social Isolation: Self-perceived Problems of a Group of Multiple Sclerosis Sufferers*. Health Services Unit Report No. 27. Canterbury: University of Kent.
2. Burnfield, A., Burnfield P. (1978). Common psychological problems in multiple sclerosis. *British Medical Journal*; **1**:1193.
3. Lloyd G. (1977). Psychological reactions to physical illness. *British Journal of Hospital Medicine*; 352.
4. Bacon, Francis (1972). *Essay XXX: On Regiment of Health*. London: J.M. Dent & Sons.
5. Burnfield A. (1977). Multiple sclerosis: a doctor's personal experience. *British Medical Journal*: **1**:435.
6. Hartings, M., Pavlou M., Davis F. (1976). Group counselling of MS patients in a program of comprehensive care. *Journal of Chronic Diseases*; **29**:65.

The Family Reaction

John Larberg and Pam Cavallo are social workers involved with The Patient Services Program in New York (of which John Larberg is Head)

This chapter is written from the American viewpoint, but its conclusions are equally valid in many Western communities. The first part of the chapter deals with the structure and functions of the family unit of modern times and then goes on to look at the influences — political, financial and social — prevalent in the USA today and how these have affected the structure of its society in general, and families in particular.

Bearing these influences in mind, the authors then consider their effects on people with MS and their families, and the needs and problems of these people living in American society today.

It is a truism that all human relationships are complex. The more intimate they are, the more complex and demanding they become. Merely holding and maintaining them requires effort and energy; for them to flourish and grow, even under the best of circumstances, the partners or participants must invest a major portion of their emotional capital, as well as their thought, their time and even their physical effort. And what set of relationships is more intimate than those in the primary unit, the family? Stresses and strains push and pull at all the family members and stretch the ties that bind—even under ideal conditions.

Then, add to this 'normally' stressful human condition the extraordinarily stressful circumstance of MS. One partner or member, probably a spouse and parent, suffers the impact of this frequently debilitating, often progressive, always unpredictable neurological disease of unknown origin, incurable and untreatable. For most, adulthood has already been achieved and major life-patterns such as career lines have been established. Very frequently, spouses have been chosen and often young children are present, before the MS is diagnosed. The impact can be overwhelming — multiple sclerosis redefines one's life and the lives of *all* those nearest and dearest.

This chapter has been written in an attempt to describe this impact and some of its potential ramifications, based on knowledge of MS, on experience with MS persons and others who deal with them almost daily, and on a perception of the many cultural and social influences surrounding them. Of necessity, this perspective is biased— biased not only by the authors' experience with MS and their profession, but biased by the fact that they live and work in the USA. The USA, then, is the context for these observations and judgements and readers from other countries will need to review their own experiences for comparisons of pertinent similarities and differences.

The MS person and family live in the context provided by their community in the broadest sense— their neighbourhood, their nation and their culture. Trends and events in the wide world outside the family affect the family as well as the surrounding community.

THE MODERN FAMILY

A word about the family as a unit of social organisation in modern times may be in order. The older, more traditional definition of the family, a married couple with a child or children, is currently undergoing a change. According to the US Bureau of Labor Statistics, this way of life represents a minority of only 40% of the households in the USA. Ann Hartman[1] proposes that the family be redefined as comprising two or more individuals who define themselves as a family and who, over time, assume those obligations toward one another that are generally considered essential components of family systems.

One can discern a trend. Many observers have noted a lessening of the importance of the role of the family paralleling the growth of industrialisation and urbanisation. The family— once defined to include not only two, but at least three generations and, in 'simpler' cultures, an extended clan of lateral kinship ties — once was not only the source of one's identity and one's values and beliefs, but also the responsible social unit for all manner of acculturation, education and training.

As social organisation has become more complex, the fulfilling of various social functions has become more and more specialised and a variety of other institutions has been born which have grown to considerable size. Many of the functions that were formerly assumed to be part of the role of the traditional family have been assigned to these institutions. Thus, we have the development of churches and synagogues, schools, training institutions, universities; in fact, businesses, governmental agencies— the whole array of organisations that have been created to accomplish narrower and specifically defined ends. This is also clearly so in such specialised functions as recreation, social welfare and public health. As a consequence, increasingly the need for the family to provide for each individual member has been lessened in many areas.

In most countries we now observe a family unit that is more narrowly defined and to which is ascribed a more circumscribed role. However, that is not to say that the family is a social unit which is no longer necessary and which other social inventions will replace completely. In fact, in the previously quoted article by Hartman, she also states: 'The family is a remarkably enduring institution, which continues to be the primary provider of help to individuals. In spite of the forecasts of breakdown, the family still provides the lion's share of health care in this country.' The family is still the essential social unit for all societies around the world, perhaps more dominant in some cultures than others. It is also still the unit through which our earliest learning and values are acquired and is still our primary source of identity.

THE FAMILY IN SOCIETY

What then are some of the modern events and trends which can be discerned to have an impact on the family and which therefore should influence the way one views the family with a member who has MS?

The thesis of this chapter asserts that a multitude of events are having an impact on the modern family and that some of the consequences are yet to be fully understood and worked out. In the USA, the rate of change and the powerful effect of those changes on society at large, and then on the family as a unit, have been truly astonishing in the past decade or two. Clearly, basic assumptions and some of our most cherished beliefs have been and are being challenged by these changes. A discussion of a few of these should provide a broader context for the understanding of MS in the family.

Limits on 'the American Dream'

The recent energy shortage in the USA has been a major element in further underscoring a shift in the American consciousness and a growing awareness of the need to examine basic assumptions about growth and development under which this society has operated. The public is increasingly aware of finite resources; of the loss of the great frontier; of limits that are now being placed on 'the American dream'. In the past five to ten years, many people have been discovering a need to think in terms of 'zero population growth' and to consider profoundly the implications of earlier traditions of wide open spaces; of 'the land of opportunity' ready to be exploited for the benefit of human beings moving across a continent. What is the implication of this shift in expectations and of the concept of sharing resources and the community's wealth and potential, as the slices of the pie get smaller because the pie itself can no longer be expected to grow ad infinitum?

Working Women and Women's Liberation

There have been significant changes in the American work force. The percentage of women who enter the work force alongside men has grown with each decennial census, to a point where now we have upwards of 75% American adult women in the work force. What impact has this had on the family as a unit?

In the USA, there is an increasingly visible and influential women's liberation movement. As women become liberated from their previously prescribed and proscribed roles in society, relationships between individual men and women in the community and in the family have begun to shift. The working out of these relationships and new role expectations continues.

Role of Government: Responsibility and Credibility

There have been changes also in the public's understanding of the role of government. Depending upon which expert or observer one listens to, the so-called credibility gap between the public and its government has created great problems of governance and has had a remarkable influence on the thinking of governmental leaders and politicans in this country. One consequence of this realisation has been a corollary that fewer people believe that government can, or perhaps even should, solve their problems. Communities, organisations, agencies, and ordinary citizens are increasingly hearing and seem to be believing that individuals and their families should be the source of their support; government should then be less involved in their affairs, not only in terms of regulating and ordering the behaviour of citizens, but also in terms of providing basic supports for citizens in trouble.

This would represent a reversal of trend. A look at the social and health insurance programmes in the USA would reveal a gradual but perceptive increase. From the worldwide depression of the 1930s to a point in the late 1970s, the growth of federal funding and programming for social and health needs of individuals, families and communities was considerable. The combined budget of the Departments of Health and Human Services and Education (formerly the Department of Health, Education and Welfare) had achieved the dominant role in the budget of the federal government, exceeding the expenditures for armaments and defence.

Our international readers should understand that there has never yet been in this country a national health scheme closely approximating those that exist in many western European nations. The programme that has existed in the USA has been heavily built on the existing 'fee for service' system of delivery of medicine and the bolstering and supporting of previously existing medical institutions in this country. The exact future of the changes as proposed by President Reagan are not clear, but the main thrust is one of, yet again, a vast and profound change in the role of government; and this in turn will cause a significant shift in thinking and expectations on the part of individuals and families who in the past have come to depend upon their government to provide a major support in their times of need.

Financial Support Systems

The plan of the Reagan Administration is to change the previous financial support structures and to reduce the amount of federal funding. By the use of 'block grants' to the states, the decision on the expenditure of the remaining funds for various competing programmes (e.g. child welfare, community development, programmes for the ageing, health, etc.) will require perhaps an extended period of struggle and will have as yet untold but predictably far-reaching consequences.

This political turn to the right in the USA with its return to an emphasis on 'rugged individualism' and the reliance on the private non-governmental sector both economically and socially, will become a phenomenon in all social and health planning and in all family considerations. This will have an obvious special meaning to persons who are the most vulnerable in society— persons with chronic ill-health, whose self-support is questionable and whose very survival has been threatened.

The Youth Culture

There are a number of cultural trends that continue to have a peculiar impact on the thinking of individuals and on the relationships in families. We can speak of the adulation of youth in the USA reinforced by sexual symbolism in all manner of publications and by the media of entertainment and communication, as well as countless advertisements to encourage the sale of products and services. It is hard to measure objectively the influence of this prevailing cultural phenomenon, but it certainly is part of the context in which all families must exist.

Money, Drugs, Crime, the 'Me Generation'

What can be said of a society in which money is seen as the primary measure of success? What is the implication of the growth of the so-called drug culture in urban, suburban, and even rural or semi-rural America?

Many commentators — religious, sociological and others — observe the loosening of the social compact and an erosion of the bonds that hold communities together; as the institutions in society that had been expected to provide support for families and to help keep them intact are themselves confronted by threats to their continuing existence and their viability. The growth of both white-collar crime and crimes of violence throughout communities is seen by many as a symbol of the loss of trust and of the disintegration of the adhesion that once held families and communities together.

What is the true meaning of the so-called me generation, where individuals seem to be saying increasingly that they wish to make sure that they get their share of 'what's out there' and are less concerned about participating with others in sharing or togetherness? What does this do to one's sense of community?

A POSITIVE RESPONSE

On the other hand, it is not all bleak and not all of the trends are towards violence and negativism. Another important facet of the last decade has been an increasing emphasis on consumerism and on neighbourhood and community participation. Americans across the USA were inspired and lifted up by the response of the great city of New York to threats to its fiscal stability and its very survival. Faced with possible bankruptcy and serious crises in programme funding, individuals, families and neighbourhoods rose to the challenge and began to lend a hand to maintain and improve the quality of life in the city. Run-down buildings have been restored and renewed by voluntary effort. Community projects of many kinds have grown up. Small garden plots have appeared; murals have been painted on blank building walls. Crossing guards, volunteers in schools, tutors and aides have emerged. Imaginative programmes have grown where individuals have said, in effect: 'We want to keep our city. We want to keep it alive and we will show that we can make a difference!'

There appears to have been also a discernible return on the part of many to religious and cultural values they previously may have felt were passé or out of style and fashion. In the newspapers and on television programmes in the USA, there are not infrequently human interest stories revealing the dedication of individuals to community values, to the needs of their friends and their families, even in the face of extremely adverse circumstances. Churches and ethical groups have raised their voices in protest against what they see as the unbridled greed of corporations and have begun to have an impact not only on the conservation of natural resources, but are also beginning to hold elected political representatives to account for the trust placed in them.

SOME IMPLICATIONS

What has been described up to this point is a society undergoing increasingly rapid change, where values and concepts once believed to be immutable and unchanging are being called into question. This has had an effect, in the USA at least, in almost every sector and every phase of modern life. The challenges to categorical thinking or prejudgements abound on all sides: civil rights movements, women's liberation, gay liberation; consumerism; the questioning of the power and the size of government, of major corporations, even of labour unions have continued apace. The so-called sexual revolution of the 1960s has enabled people to seek new ways to express their own innermost needs in a socially positive and acceptable fashion, even though unconventionally in some instances.

All of these social, economic, cultural, educational and other events and trends have a direct bearing on the strength and viability of family units in our society. For a family to survive it must develop new coping mechanisms. It must find a balance between steadiness and flexibility, and must know where and how to adapt itself to the winds of change.

This, then, is the context for families in the USA, impressionistically stated. As we now turn to the special impact of multiple sclerosis on the family, one can have a keener appreciation of the challenge of living and coping daily with this unpredictable and terrible disease.

As noted earlier, most persons with MS are increasingly assuming many social and economic responsibilities. The initial impact is likely to occur when they are just in the beginning or middle of things. Multiple sclerosis is not like other diseases. It is ambiguous, uncertain and uncontrollable. It is an unexpected blow for which no one is ever prepared; and certainly no one is prepared for the unique stress it imposes.

Joan Didion, the well known American author, describes the impact and uncertainty of MS in her book, *The White Album*:[2]

> I had, at this time, a sharp apprehension not of what it was like to be old but of what it was like to open the door to the stranger and find

> that the stranger did indeed have the knife. In a few lines of dialogue in a neurologist's office in Beverly Hills, the improbable had become the probable, the norm: things which happened only to other people could in fact happen to me. I could be struck by lightning, could dare to eat a peach and be poisoned by the cyanide in the stone . . . in other words—it was another story without narrative . . . I was told that the disorder was not really in my eyes, but in my central nervous system. I might or might not experience symptoms of neural damage all my life. These symptoms, which might or might not appear, might or might not involve my eyes. They might or might not involve my arms or legs, they might or might not be disabling. Their effects might be lessened by cortisone injections, or they might not. It could not be predicted. The condition had a name, the kind of name usually associated with telethons, but the name was multiple sclerosis, but the name had no meaning. This was, the neurologist said, an exclusionary diagnosis, and meant nothing.

Illness is truly the night-side of life and society's attitudes concerning illness and disease serve to blacken the night needlessly. Susan Sontag, in *Illness as a Metaphor*,[3] analyses the modern predilection for psychological explanations of disease. The meaning of illness and disease has been greatly influenced by the emphasis on psychological aspects of behaviour. People are encouraged to believe that they get sick because they unconsciously want to; they are encouraged to believe that their personality causes disease because it is either deficient or has not expressed itself.

Abundant metaphors concerning illness and disease can be found today in medical, psychological, social and philosophical thinking. Categories which were developed to describe those people whose personalities render them likely candidates for certain diseases still exist, as for example, 'the cancer personality'. These theories are punitive and a powerful means of placing the blame for illness on the sick person. Those diseases particularly prone to psychological and metaphorical interpretations are those whose causality is murky and for which treatment is largely ineffective. Hence, the metaphysical and even mythical explanations for disease.

Multiple sclerosis fits quite well into this line of thinking: its cause is unknown and treatment is ineffectual. Add the adult onset, unpredictability, an erratic course, difficulty in establishing a diagnosis and varying complexes of symptomatology and invisible symptoms, such as blurred vision and fatigue. Unfortunately, because of this, psychological explanations persist and undermine the 'reality' of the disease and weaken the ability of MS persons and families to understand the illness and what is happening to them.

The need exists to combat these theories and establish the 'reality' of the illness. Peyser *et al.*[4] made such a contribution in an article which describes a preliminary investigation of MS patients' psychological profiles: 'We believe that past attempts to delineate a specific MS personality have failed for the reason that it would be naive to expect that all patients, regardless of their unique personal and symptom complex, will react in the same fashion and fit into a single pattern.'

Multiple sclerosis can seriously affect a person's body, disrupt family life and work, and strain finances. It can threaten a person's sources of support, self-esteem and identification.

Social needs are created by the disease; needs for non-medical support and assistance. The greatest needs for support and assistance concern the individual's and spouse's reactions and their adjustment to the illness—the marital relationship and their children's adjustment. These findings are documented by Braham *et al.*[5] who studied the social needs of 47 non-hospitalised persons with MS. The day-to-day work of the chapters of the United States National Multiple Sclerosis Society is consistent with Braham's findings. Locally conducted surveys of needs reveal that counselling of all types for individuals with MS, their spouses and children is a frequently requested service of the National Multiple Sclerosis Society Chapters.

'It's not true, it can't happen to me.' Denial is a frequent initial response to the disease. Matson and Brooks[6] maintain that a general process of adjustment is fully achieved by many persons with MS. These authors, as a result of their research, have proposed a model of long-term adjustment to progressive, potentially disabling, unpredictable, but not generally fatal disease.

Denial is the first stage in this model, with resistance second: 'It won't get me down!' Affirmation is the third stage: 'I guess I have to face it'; and integration the fourth: 'I know it's there, but I don't think much about it'. Individuals may not follow the stages of the model in the order given; nor does everyone progress through all stages. They may regress to a previous stage or remain in one stage in this process, if the disease stabilises.

Isolation and inactivity are potential, and all too often actual, results of chronic illness. The need for human connections continues when a person becomes ill. As Germain writes:[1] 'In a human being, relatedness is both a biological and psychological imperative. Caring for and being cared for are deeply felt human needs as long as life lasts.' Yet, chronic illness frequently limits and sometimes cuts off opportunities for human contact.

Damaged self-image and self-esteem are a problem related to loss of physical function and activity restriction. Indeed, Matson and Brooks found that their subjects' self-concept decreased as the disease brought on greater impairment and restrictions.

How does a person cope? What helps a person get through? Religion and the family were found, in one study, to be the most frequently used coping strategies.[6]

Religion, by its nature, provides a foundation for living; but the family itself is seriously affected by the disease. While each family style and situation is different, a core experience has been identified by Pavlou *et al.*,[7] called 'family pain'. This is the hurt experienced by the entire group in response to this misfortune in one of its members. The family members may feel fear and anger. They feel powerless in face of the disease and feel they should make the MS family member happy or make up for this terrible situation. Sometimes, 'family pain' appears not only as anger but also as bitterness, lack of caring and insensitivity.

Common issues identified by Pavlou *et al.* are a result of their projects and ongoing programme of comprehensive care at the Multiple Sclerosis Center, Rush Presbyterian, St Lukes Medical Center, Chicago, Illinois. The following are concerns and difficulties expressed by MS family members.

- Wondering how much to assist the patient, and how much to push the patient to function independently; wondering if the patient could be doing more for himself or herself.
- Confused by fluctuations in the disease— why can the patient do so much more some days than others— what problems are related to MS and which are not, and are all disabilities 'legitimate'?
- Feeling burdened by the patient's depression or irritability.
- Worried about whether there will be a proper environment for children getting MS.
- Concern that marital partners cannot talk about MS together — partners disguise thoughts in an attempt to protect each other.
- Exhausted by having to assume extra responsibilities, and resentment that it is assumed that they can handle everything.
- Belief that the MS patient could try harder.
- Wanting the patient to make an exhaustive search for a cure.
- Family becoming disorganised by overwhelming physical care need and unable to get outside help.
- Not talking about the problem and hoping that maybe it will go away.
- Problems with the extended family— everyone has different ideas

about what should be done, and everyone criticises what everyone else is doing (translation: everyone feels guilty).

Other feelings are also stated, but less easily. They are less 'socially acceptable'. They include the following.

- Feeling obligated or trapped. Nearly universally, a family member thinks of leaving, sometimes with a fleeting question of what it would be like, and sometimes with a more frank wish for separation or divorce. The spouse often feels less free, simply because of the fact of the disease, and feels obligated and resentful on these grounds alone.
- Missing recreational pastimes, now closed to the family because of MS.
- Feeling embarrassed by the MS person, particularly in public. This feeling is not readily acknowledged, but is expressed sometimes by young adolescent children. They wonder what to tell friends about the MS patient.
- Being simply tired of living with MS night and day.
- Wishing for care themselves.
- Feeling burdened by perpetual responsibility for making special arrangements, particularly when the family goes out.[7]

Placed in the overall context described earlier, it can be said that there are several nodal points for adjustment and readjustment to MS. We propose the following nine points, each of which may make the family particularly vulnerable and in need of outside counselling or other help.

1. The point of receiving the MS diagnosis (regardless of the degree of progression or disablement).
2. Any exacerbation.
3. Any residual loss of function, however gradual.
4. Specifically, loss of mobility.
5. Loss of bladder or bowel function.
6. Loss of 'normal' sexual function.
7. Loss of job or status.
8. At the time of severe physical dependency.
9. Possible loss of spouse or other significant relationships.

Many families manage well with MS. But, just as the person with MS needs support and assistance, so too the family needs support and assistance. Mary Richmond wrote:[1] 'The beneficial results of individual treatment would "crumble away if workers failed to take account of the family".'

REFERENCES

1. Hartmann Ann (1981). The family: a central focus for practice. *Journal of Social Work*; **26**(1).
2. Didion Joan (1979). *The White Album*. New York: Simon and Schuster.
3. Sontag S. (1974). *Illness as a Metaphor*.
4. Peyser J.M. *et al*. (1980). Psychological profiles in patients with multiple sclerosis. *Archives of Neurology*; **37**:437.
5. Braham Sara *et al*. (1975). Evaluation of the social needs of nonhospitalised chronically ill persons. *Journal of Chronic Diseases*; **28**.
6. Matson R.R., Brooks N.A. (1977). Adjusting to multiple sclerosis: an exploratory study. *Social Science and Medicine*; **11**:245.
7. Pavlou J.M. *et al*. (1979). A program of psychologic service delivery in a multiple sclerosis center. *Professional Psychology*.

Sexual Implications of Multiple Sclerosis

Michael Barrett is Associate Professor in Zoology at the University of Toronto, Canada, and Chairperson of the Sex Information and Education Council of Canada.

In this chapter, he begins by giving an account of the physiology of sexual responses in both men and women and then goes on to relate the ways in which these responses can differ in those suffering from MS. The chapter is well referenced to allow those who are interested to obtain details of current and past research into the subject.

The effects of altered sexual response are discussed, as are the possible reasons— psychogenic and neurogenic— for these alterations. The chapter suggests ways of dealing with various dysfunctions and associated problems and reviews some sexual side-effects of medications for MS, as well as the subjects of fertility and contraception as they relate to people with MS.

It is hoped that an understanding of the sexual implications of the disease and the knowledge that it does not lead to an end to sexual pleasure will help both those suffering from it and the people involved with them to cope with the changes it may produce.

The neurological damage associated with MS can have a direct effect on the physiology of sexual response. In men, the effects can include: difficulty in getting or maintaining an erection; partial erection that is lost during intercourse; ejaculation that occurs much more quickly or more slowly than was previously the case; lack of orgasm; reduced force of ejaculation. In addition numbness or lack of sensation in the genitals may impede sexual responsiveness and muscle spasms; and physical weakness or lack of mobility may force changes in previously established patterns of sexual interaction.[1,2]

The neurological mechanisms controlling sexual response appear to be similar in both sexes and women may therefore experience changes comparable to those described for men. These can include: lack of vaginal lubrication or clitoral engorgement; difficulty in achieving orgasm; genital insensitivity with resulting lack of response to either clitoral or vaginal stimulation; hypersensitivity that makes genital stimulation unpleasant or, at times, painful; adductor spasms that interfere with sexual intercourse; lack of muscle strength necessitating changed positioning for sexual activity; pain during sexual intercourse.

While these symptoms may increase in severity and frequency as the disease progresses, it is not uncommon to find changes in sexual response in people who are not severely handicapped. Variability between individuals and within the same person over time can make it difficult to predict these changes or to interpret their origins easily when they do occur. This last point is a real concern for professionals working with people who have MS. While the symptoms described above can and do arise as a direct consequence of nerve damage associated with the disease, they can also arise indirectly as a result of psychological or relational reactions to MS. The *interaction* between neurological factors, which might alter some aspect of sexual response, and inter- and intrapersonal factors, which govern how people cope with such alterations, are perhaps the most important elements in recognising and dealing with the sexual implications of MS.

The first part of this chapter will review what is known about the effects of MS on the physiology of sexual response. The focus will be, of necessity, on genital response and the physiological mechanisms involved in sexual arousal. Since the body of literature in this area is scant, inferences will be drawn from the more abundant literature on sexual response following spinal-cord injury.

In the second section, the problem of diagnosis will be considered. How can one tell whether the lack of erection in a man with MS is the result of neurological deficit, or of 'performance anxiety' nourished by an earlier 'failure' unrelated to but now blamed on the MS, or a combination of both? Is it necessary to make such diagnostic decisions before the person can be helped to deal with the situation?

In the last section, some corollary issues associated with sexuality and MS will be considered, including: implications of altered bowel and bladder function; sexual side-effects of commonly used medications; fertility; hormonal factors in sexual interest and responsiveness. Issues involved in counselling about sexuality and MS will be discussed elsewhere.

PHYSIOLOGY OF SEXUAL RESPONSE

Masters and Johnson[3] have provided the most widely popularised description of physical changes associated with sexual response in men and women. The phases in the sexual response cycle— excitement, plateau, orgasm and resolution — provide a convenient frame of reference in which to localise anatomical events, both genital and extragenital, associated with sexual arousal and orgasm. Their discussion of nipple erection, sex flush, rectal sphincter contractions and increased breathing rate, heart rate, blood pressure and perspiration showed that sexual response involves more than the genitals. Genital responsiveness is nevertheless an important feature of sexual arousal, and an understanding of the mechanisms involved in genital sexual response in able-bodied men and women is the first step in understanding how these mechanisms can be affected by MS.

Recent research, much of it done in relation to spinal-cord-injured men and women, has expanded our knowledge of the neurophysiology of sexual response.[4–10] The discussion that follows will draw heavily on Geiger's analysis of the neurological control of sexual response.[10]

SEXUAL RESPONSE IN MEN

Sexual response involves two physiological phenomena: *myotonia* (increased muscle tension) and *vasocongestion* (in which blood flows more rapidly into than it does out of a particular region). These changes are mediated by the involuntary (autonomic) nervous system but to some extent by the somatic system as well.

Erection

Erection is the first sign of sexual arousal in men. Dilatation of blood vessels supplying the corpora of the penis (two regions of spongy tissue, the corpora cavernosa, lie above the urethra and a third, the corpus spongiosum, surrounds the urethra and swells at the end of the penis to form the glans) causes blood to flow into these areas faster than it flows out. The result is engorgement and erection.

Dilatation of the blood vessels can occur either *psychogenically*, as a result of the mental stimulation of dreams, fantasy, memory or the sight, smell, sound or taste of a partner (or other erotic cue), or *reflexogenically*, as a result of either direct external genital (or perineal) stimulation or internal reflex stimulation such as that caused by a full bladder. Reflexogenic erection could occur as follows. Physical caressing of the penis sends impulses along the dorsal nerve of the penis to the pudendal nerve which carries the information to the sacral (S_2–S_4) region of the spinal cord. The sensory fibres of the pudendal nerve synapse with motor fibres of the parasympathetic nervous system which send impulses back along the pelvic nerve, to cause dilatation of blood vessels, and along the pudendal nerve (part of the somatic nervous system) to cause contraction of the bulbocavernosus and ischiocavernosus muscles. These contractions allow blood which would normally have been shunted into outgoing veins to flow into the penis instead, thus further facilitating erection.

Psychogenic erection occurs when impulses from the brain, presumably initiated by erotic awareness, travel down the spinal cord in fibres that synapse with sympathetic nervous system ganglia at the 11th thoracic to 2nd lumbar levels (T_{11}–L_2). Postganglionic fibres at this level carry impulses to cause dilatation of penile blood vessels. These impulses, originating in the brain, probably travel to the sacral region of the cord where parasympathetic fibres of the pelvic nerve may also participate to induce erection.

Usually the reflex and psychogenic mechanisms occur concurrently. Indeed, both must usually be operating for erection to be maintained. Any extended interruption of physical input or inhibition of psychogenic input (e.g. anxiety, distraction) can, as Geiger puts it,[10] 'be devastating to the best erection!'.

Ejaculation

The terms ejaculation and orgasm are often used interchangeably, although the former is a 'pelvic' and the latter an essentially 'cerebral' event. It is possible for a man to ejaculate without experiencing the sensation of orgasm, and *vice versa*. Thus, although the two phenomena usually occur together, they might better be viewed as separate entities from a neurological standpoint.

Physiologically, ejaculation itself involves two processes. The first, *emission*, involves rhythmic smooth muscle contraction in the seminal vesicles, vas deferens and prostate gland. This process releases semen into the prostatic urethra and is mediated by sympathetic nerves exiting in the T_{11}–L_2 region of the spinal cord. This may be the source of the feeling of 'ejaculatory inevitability' described by Masters and Johnson.[3]

The second process, *ejaculation*, involves contraction of bulbocavernosus and ischiocavernosus muscles plus other muscles of the pelvic floor and causes expulsion of semen from the prostatic urethra. This aspect of the process is mediated by the somatic nervous system via motor fibres originating in the sacral (S_2–S_4) segments of the cord and carried in the pudendal nerve to striated muscle in the pelvis. At the same time, sympathetic fibres from the T_{12}–L_2 region cause contraction of the neck of the bladder so that semen is expelled to the outside rather than back into the bladder. Retrograde ejaculation occurs when semen is pushed back into the bladder as a result of the inability of the sympathetic nervous system, either due to nerve damage or bladder neck resection, to close the neck of the bladder.

Orgasm

The subjective experience of orgasm usually occurs concurrently with the pelvic events of ejaculation. Impulses from the genitals to the limbic system in the brain bring awareness of the sensations and the feeling of release of tension. At the time of orgasm there are also a number of extragenital changes including: anal sphincter contractions; specific skeletal muscle contractions; hyperventilation; increased heart rate.[3] Although it is often assumed that the experience of orgasm occurs *as a result* of the brain's perception of genital sensations during ejaculation, it seems likely that men can experience orgasm even when the nervous connection between brain and genitals has been severed, as in spinal-cord injury.[10] The use of the term 'phantom orgasm' to describe this phenomenon in cord-injured men[11] is considered a misnomer by Geiger,[10] who implies that the term diminishes an experience that is real for those who may describe it variously as a warm sensation, severe muscular spasticity, physical pleasure, sexual excitation or even headache.[12]

Cohen *et al.*[13] note that the focus of earlier research on the changes in the autonomic nervous system and peripheral musculature at orgasm has given us 'a peripherally focused account of the process of sexual climax, in which blood flow changes and muscular contractions are commonly viewed as the crucial determinants of human orgasm'. They observed statistically significant changes in laterality of left and right parietal EEGs in men and women at climax and concluded that: 'future models of human sexual response will need to incorporate brain phenomena associated with orgasm'. This would include the possibility that men who lack genital sensitivity or response could learn to 'eroticise' non-genital stimulation and to experience a sense of tension release following a period of sustained stimulation. Higgins[12] recognises this as an interesting and little understood area for future research and emphasises, as have other authors, our limited understanding of the neurological aspects of orgasm.

SEXUAL RESPONSE IN WOMEN

The sexual response cycle in women has physiological parallels to the most obviously emphasised events in male sexual response (erection and ejaculation) and is mediated in the pelvis by the same nerves as in the male. According to Geiger,[10] these consist of 'fibres from the lowest sympathetic ganglia, the presacral parasympathetics and sensory and motor fibres of the pudendal nerve'. The changes that occur during sexual response can be summarised using the Masters and Johnson terminology of the four phases.

Excitement

Vasocongestion in the pelvis as a result of either reflex or psychogenic stimulation causes vaginal lubrication, engorgement of the labia and engorgement of the clitoris. The vaginal barrel begins to lengthen and distend and the uterus to elevate. In addition, nipple erection, the beginning of breast engorgement, and increases in respiration, pulse and blood pressure occur. Men also experience most of these extragenital changes but have been less encouraged to focus on them as aspects of sexual response.

Plateau

The vaginal barrel continues to increase in length and as the inner two-thirds dilates the outer one-third becomes more fully engorged to form, together with the engorged labia minora, the so-called orgasmic platform.[3] During this phase, the clitoris retracts, the areola become engorged with blood (in some cases giving the impression that nipple erection has disappeared) and increased blood flow to the skin gives rise, in some women, to a 'sex flush'. In addition, increased build-up in voluntary and involuntary muscle contraction plus further elevation of the uterus set the stage for release of sexual tension in orgasm.

Orgasm

Physiological events at orgasm include rhythmic contractions of the 'orgasmic platform', of the uterus and of the anal sphincter, coupled with increased skeletal muscle tension, and peaks in blood pressure, pulse rate and respiration rate. These all have their physiological parallels in male orgasm and are thought to be similarly mediated.

Some women are able to achieve orgasm from fantasy or nipple stimulation alone, suggesting that orgasm is not dependent on direct genital stimulation. However, since their genitals undergo changes similar to those experienced by women during intercourse or manual clitoral stimulation, it may be that their mental experience of orgasm comes in part from the perceived sensation of the genital changes described above. However, descriptions of orgasm by spinal-cord-injured women[14] suggest that physical and psychological feelings of sexual climax can occur even in the absence of perceived genital sensation. This observation has relevance to people with any type of neurological impairment and highlights the importance of the previously discussed distinction between ejaculation and orgasm.

Resolution

This phase involves the gradual reversal of changes that occurred during excitement and plateau, during which pelvic organs and other tissues that became engorged with blood are restored to their unstimulated condition. This also occurs in men. One difference, however, is the ability of some women to have several orgasms in succession. Men generally have a latent or refractory period after ejaculation, the duration varying from man to man, and only after that time has passed can they be restimulated to plateau phase levels of arousal and another ejaculation.

EFFECTS OF MS ON SEXUAL FUNCTIONING IN MEN

Only a few research studies have examined the sexual implications of MS. These have focused, not surprisingly, on ability to have erection, to have sexual intercourse and to experience ejaculation. Ivers and Goldstein[15] reported that 26% of their male patients were impotent and that for 3% it was the principal symptom of the disease. Vas[16] found that 47% of a sample of 37 men with MS (age 18–50; mean = 39 years) were partially or totally impotent. He described impotence as 'a disturbance of sexual function in the male that precluded satisfactory coitus' and considered it *partial* in the case of 'an inability to attain or maintain full erection' and *total* if there was 'total loss of erective prowess'. These distinctions appear to correlate with other functional differences. For example, abnormalities of sensation and of bowel and bladder function were more common in the totally impotent men than in those described as partially impotent or normally potent. Similarly, the totally impotent men complained more frequently of incontinence or urine retention than did those in the other two groups, and the partially impotent men were more likely to report urgency or urinary incontinence than were their normally potent counterparts. This association between erectile dysfunction and disturbance of other autonomically controlled functions suggests a neurological rather than psychological basis for altered erectile capacity. Indeed, Vas[16] showed that the three totally impotent men in his study lacked scrotal, bulbocavernosus and cremasteric reflexes. These reflexes were intact in the majority of normally potent patients and were more frequently abnormal in the partially impotent men. More will be said later about the problem of distinguishing between neurogenic and psychogenic impotence. Vas's findings suggest that the lesions associated with MS are of the 'upper motor neuron' type and that disturbances of sexual response in MS are similar in some respects to those seen in other conditions involving upper motor neuron lesions.[5]

It is worth noting that Vas selected for his study only men who were not severely disabled. Thus men who required a cane to walk or who were unable to work or continue their normal activities of living were not investigated. This suggests that altered patterns of sexual response may be early symptoms of MS and that they can occur in the absence of severe disability.

While Vas used the term 'impotence' in a 'clinical' way, some authors have suggested that it should be discarded, along with terms such as 'frigid', because of the unwarranted connotations it carries.[17] Men with MS who are unable to have erections may nevertheless be sexually active, erotically attractive and agreeable to their partners, and socially and professionally competent. The label 'impotent' appears to deny these potential qualities and is therefore needlessly stigmatising and misleading. This is not to say that men with MS may not feel the stigma of this label, or even apply it to themselves if they experience the symptom. Altered sexual response can be devastating to the self-esteem of some men and a source of anxiety and uncertainty for their partners. Insightful counselling under such circumstances is essential for both partners and is an important professional responsibility for those in the helping professions. Issues involved in sex counselling for people with MS will be explored elsewhere, but it should be emphasised that lack of erection does not mean lack of sexual interest or libido. Vas noted that all of the men in his study 'apparently had normal libidinous desires'.

As MS symptoms worsen, one might expect changes in sexual interest, enjoyment and activity to become more apparent. For example, in a study of 115 men aged 17–60, it was found that only 9% considered their sex lives to be unchanged 'in general', whereas 64% found it either unsatisfactory or 'finished'.[18] The nature of the changes included the following: 56% considered their interest in sexual intercourse to be either decreased or finished; satisfaction with and frequency of intercourse were similarly altered; and 80% reported either decreased (50%) or finished (30%) erection. These men were more severely disabled than the population studied by Vas[16] and had a higher incidence of complaints associated with what they described as unsatisfactory or finished sexual lives. Among the 75 men who identified their sexual lives in this way, the most frequently cited 'main problems' were: loss of erection (64%); weak erection (12%); weakness of body muscles (12%); spasticity (10.7%); 'frigidity' of wife (8%); periodical loss of erection (6.7%); premature ejaculation (5.3%).

Another report on a sample of 25 men with MS, showed that 32% had decreased libido, 44% had difficulty in achieving erection, 44% had retarded or absent ejaculation, and 52% had 'orgasmic troubles'.[19] Burnfield[20] attests to the frequent occurrence of erectile dysfunction in men with MS and also cites Miller *et al.*[21] who found this symptom in 60% of MS patients. Burnfield wisely points out that 'impotence' does occur in the general population; that it can have psychogenic origins and reinforcements; and that 'potency problems can relapse and remit like any other symptom of MS'. She warns against dismissing patients' concerns with the simple admonition: 'It's all part of MS, you'll have to learn to live with it.' Unfortunately, men have been encouraged to focus on penile erection and 'performance' in intercourse as the primary, perhaps even exclusive, definers of their sexuality. Much of the literature on male sexuality and MS reflects this preoccupation. The intra- and interpersonal issues arising from the erectile dysfunction, be it psychogenic or neurogenic, are equally important,[20, 22, 23, 24] but less frequently discussed with people who have MS.

EFFECT OF MS ON SEXUAL FUNCTIONING IN WOMEN

I know of only two large studies on the sexual functioning of women with MS. Lundberg[2] summarises the results of a study involving 25 women aged 20–42 (mean 31.1 years) who were clearly diagnosed as having MS but whose 'handicap score' (grade 1–2 on a 6-grade scale) indicated 'rather mild cases with slight or no disability'. They were questioned about sexual symptoms and bowel and bladder function and their responses were compared to those of a matched control group of migraine sufferers.

Among the women with MS: 36% reported difficulty in achieving orgasm; 20% had pain during intercourse; 12% described lack of vaginal lubrication; and 12% had severe dysaesthesia that, at times, made direct genital stimulation uncomfortable or unbearable. Of the women who reported some kind of sexual problem (52%), none had experienced such difficulties before the onset of MS and most said the sexual symptoms had appeared rather abruptly. In addition, 68% of the women were presently experiencing or had a history of urinary troubles, e.g. urgency, incontinence, or slight urinary retention, and 48% reported past or present constipation (and, in two cases, some bowel incontinence as well). Sexual dysfunction was rare in the control group and acute loss of libido, genital paraesthesiae or incontinence was not reported at all. These findings suggest that the sexual symptoms were a direct result of the neurological effects of MS rather than of 'psychological' factors such as fatigue, anxiety or depression.

On neurological examination, the women with MS showed 'an obvious correlation between genital sensory symptoms and sensory signs as well as loss of sacral cord reflexes'.[25] These observations reinforce the idea of a neurologically based sexual dysfunction, although it would be important for any helping professional to examine the implications of the symptoms in the total context of the woman's relationships, self-image and lifestyle.

Lundberg[2] points out that some of the women were able to achieve orgasm despite 'fairly intense sensory symptoms', and that all but one of the women continued to have intercourse, although at a diminished frequency in most cases. The one woman who had stopped having intercourse experienced vaginismus. Although Lundberg does not say so, it is possible that this involuntary vaginal closure in response to attempted vaginal penetration originated secondarily to pain during intercourse. The pain may have come from reduced vaginal lubrication or genital dysaesthesiae, both of which can have their roots in neurological disturbances. This example shows how a change in sexual response arising from a nerve damage associated with MS might lead to a sexual dysfunction that is thought to be 'psychological' in nature. Lundberg's findings suggest that important changes in sexual response, 'most probably correlated to anatomical lesions in the central nervous system', can occur even in women having early or mild MS.

A study was made of a sample of 134 women, aged 17–60, whose symptoms were more pronounced than in the previous group and whose average age was perhaps 10 years higher (70.9% of the women were 31–50).[18] While 28% of these women considered their sexual lives to be, in general, unchanged (in contrast to 9% of the men in a study by the same authors) and 33% described them as fairly good, 39% considered their sexual lives unsatisfactory or finished. In this population, 42% said their interest in sexual intercourse was decreased or finished; 50% reported a similar status for their satisfaction with sexual intercourse; 43% said the frequency of intercourse had decreased; and 19% said it had finished; 49% noted decreased or finished clitoral sensitivity; and 57% said the same about their ability to achieve orgasm.

Of the 53 women in this group who considered their sexual lives unsatisfactory or finished, the main problems cited were: loss of orgasm (33%); loss of libido (27%); spasticity (12%); husband's refusal to engage in intercourse (9%); weakness of body muscles (9%); lack of sexual partner (5%); vaginal dryness (5%).

In addition to changes in sexual response that might be directly attributable to the neurological effects of MS, women (and men) may also experience fatigue, difficulty in communicating about sexual matters, anxiety about their partners' reactions, or other situational changes; all of which can alter sexual interest and responsiveness.[20] The net effect is that many people prematurely terminate their sexual lives or carry on in a state of unremedied dissatisfaction. Many of them could be helped by knowledgeable counselling,[20] and those who are satisfied with their sexual lives could be helped to avoid problems if they learned to recognise and adapt to possible changes in sexual response patterns before they develop into relationship-threatening dysfunctions.

DISTINGUISHING BETWEEN ORGANIC AND PSYCHOGENIC SEXUAL DYSFUNCTION

The advent of surgical treatment of impotence by implantation of penile prostheses[26–31] has raised questions about our ability to distinguish between erectile dysfunction that has its roots in psychological factors (fear of failure, anxiety, etc.) and that caused by damage to the nerves that mediate erection. A number of authors have addressed themselves to the methods involved in making such distinctions [32, 33, 34] and to the implications of this knowledge for the counselling process.[35] These issues are of particular relevance in the counselling of people with MS because of the strong evidence linking neurological impairment with sexual dysfunction in this condition. It has been suggested that impotence associated with MS, 'when not psychogenically determined', may be due either to upper motor neuron lesions in the brainstem or above the lumbar region of the spinal cord (these block psychogenic erection) or to lower motor neuron lesions interfering with reflex erection.[1] It has also been hypothesised that lesions producing impotence in men with MS would be found in either the cervical (uppermost), dorsal (thoracic?) or lumbar areas of the cord.[16] Given the unpredictability of MS, is it possible to determine when erectile dysfunction is, and is not, 'psychogenically determined'?

It is known that men have regular periods of erection during sleep (nocturnal penile tumescence, NPT) and that this is less likely to occur in the face of either damage to the nerves mediating erection or other organic sources of erectile dysfunction. Changes in penile circumference can be measured plethysmographically during sleep and as a result many of the parameters of NPT in normal healthy men have now been determined.[32] The diagnostic potential of NPT has been studied as a means of differentiating between organic and psychogenic impotence.[34] The approach was to divide a group of men, none of whom had been able to achieve full erection by any means (with a partner, masturbation or fantasy) in the three months prior to assessment, into four diagnostic categories and to examine their NPT responses over two consecutive nights. The categories identified the likely source of the erectile dysfunction as: (1) *organic*: organic factors known to cause impotence were present in these subjects (complete flaccid paraplegia, etc.) and no relevant psychogenic factors were seen on psychiatric examination, (e.g. marital discord, performance anxiety, etc.); (2) *psychogenic*: no apparent organic cause but psychogenic factors severe enough to account for the onset of erectile dysfunction were present; (3) *mixed organic and psychogenic*: both types of factors were clearly present; (4) *uncertain*: neither organic nor psychogenic factors were detected. The authors report that decision criteria based on both the maximum penile circumference change during NPT and the maximum number of NPT episodes per night led to 95% diagnositc accuracy in distinguishing between organic and psychogenic impotence. They point out, however, that these results simply show the success of NPT analysis in confirming an existing diagnosis and that it remains to be validated as a diagnostic instrument.

Since a reliable, portable and inexpensive NPT monitor is now available, it has been argued that 'monitoring of NPT alone represents the basic minimum that should be performed in the evaluation of all males complaining of impotence'.[32] This would provide not only an assessment for possible surgical treatment,[33] but also a confirmation and reassurance for those men experiencing psychogenic impotence who are reluctant to accept the idea that their erectile dysfunction is not a 'physical' problem.[34]

In addition to monitoring of NPT, there is a variety of tests that a doctor can perform to test for reflex activity through the S_2–S_4 segments of the spinal cord and for the ability of sensations to travel from genitals to brain— or for volitional messages to go from brain to genitals.[5] These tests can be performed on both men and women and allow for some insight into the possible organic basis of sexual dysfunction. Such insights are particularly important in dealing with the sexual problems of men and women who have MS. However, the interaction of organic and psychogenic factors would be highly likely in the sexual dysfunctions associated with MS and it is therefore desirable to deal with sexual problems 'within the overall context of an individual's personal and interpersonal experience'.[35] The diagnostic tools used to differentiate between organic and psychogenic dysfunction should be seen as adjuncts to, and not substitutes for, this type of counselling.

Within the past ten years, the techniques for surgical treatment of erectile dysfunction have been developed and used with increasing frequency in the USA. Small[36] reports a high success rate with 260 implants of Silastic rods (these are inserted into the corpora of the penis and give a permanent 'semi-erection'); and Furlow[29] ascribes comparable success to a similar technique that uses inflatable prostheses which can be filled or emptied mechanically from a silicone reservoir implanted beneath the skin.

It is clear that implants are not the only way to deal with organically based erectile dysfunction. Indeed, there is some clincial evidence that 'men with diabetes or MS, whose erectile problems were assumed to be neurologically based, have regained their erectile capacity after participating in sex therapy'.[35] However, this observation may say more about the accuracy of the initial diagnosis of the problem than it does about the efficacy of different therapeutic strategies. Techniques such as NPT monitoring may provide a vehicle for resolving at least some of the uncertainty surrounding this complex area.

Women with MS may also be helped in their sexual readjustment by a clearer understanding of any obvious neurological impediments to sexual response. However, women are more likely to complain of lack of orgasm than they are of lack of vaginal lubrication (the physiological parallel in women to male erection). Given the presence of orgasmic experiences in women who have clear neurological deficits,[14] it is important to maintain an open mind about the 'orgasmic capacity' of women with MS, even those women whose neurological profiles indicate an organic basis for lost genital responsiveness. Thus, while a neurological explanation for lack of vaginal lubrication (which could be remedied through the use of K-Y jelly regardless of its origin) might also suggest the reason for lack of orgasm, it should not be taken to mean that orgasm is impossible simply because the nerve pathways for lubrication are impeded.

In summary, the methods currently available for distinguishing between 'organic' and 'psychogenic' sexual dysfunction should be approached with cautious optimism in relation to people with MS. Such distinctions can be misleading, particularly in a variable condition such as MS. More research, done specifically on people with MS, is required if we are to be freed from the need to draw inferences about MS on the basis of findings with other disabilities.

SOME OTHER IMPLICATIONS OF MS FOR SEXUAL FUNCTIONING

Bowel and Bladder Function

Since bowel and bladder are controlled via the same sacral segments that mediate sexual response, it is common, though not inevitable, to find bladder incontinence and altered sexual response together in people with MS. The reflex actions of bowel and bladder are usually controlled from the brain via nerves travelling down the spinal cord. Damage to these so-called upper motor neurons (i.e. those above the sacral region of the cord) may cause the bladder to become hyper-reflexive (over-reactive). In this situation, called 'upper motor neuron bladder', the urination reflex is no longer adequately controlled from the brain and may be set off by tapping the bladder, by rectal stimulation or by other reflex actions. This seems to be the condition that prevails in the case of MS-related incontinence.

It has been pointed out that reflex sexual response (erection or vaginal lubrication) can occur in people with upper motor neuron bladders (although ejaculation and orgasm may not), and it is suggested that counsellors who discuss bladder functioning with their clients may gain insights into sexual functioning as well.[37] In addition, 'this type of questioning may be a good lead-in for a discussion of sex'. Indeed, apprehension about incontinence during sexual activity can be both distracting and inhibiting for both partners, and counsellors should help people to deal with both the practical and attitudinal aspects of this issue. These may include: hygiene associated with catheterisation; bladder infection and ways to avoid it; preparing for sexual activity by emptying bladder and rectum; positioning of catheters; regulating fluid intake; altering positions for intercourse or other sexual activities.[38]

Sexual Side-effects of Medications

Tranquillising drugs have a depressant effect on the sympathetic nervous system and may consequently interfere with the emission and expulsion phases of ejaculation. This introduces an additional complication into our understanding of ejaculatory dysfunction in men with MS who are taking tranquillising medication. Antidepressant drugs have an indirect stimulatory effect on the sympathetic system and an inhibitory effect on the parasympathetic and may therefore interfere with erection in men and with vaginal lubrication and clitoral engorgement in women. Dominance of the sympathetic nervous system appears to inhibit arousal and facilitate ejaculation, a finding that explains, parenthetically, why anxiety may lead to either erectile dysfunction *or* 'premature' ejaculation.[39]

Some antispasmodic medications may cause a reduction of 'sex drive', a side-effect that may not be easily recognised in people with MS who may attribute any change to fatigue, stress or other symptoms of the disease. Although some drugs can clearly depress sexual interest and response (including alcohol in high doses), there are no magic potions or pills that will dramatically increase sexual interest. The supposed 'aphrodisiac' qualities of vitamin E have not been supported in research studies,[40] and the steroid sex hormone, testosterone (the presumed 'libido hormone' in both men and women), is thought to increase sex drive primarily in those who are deficient in their own production of the hormone. In this respect, it is interesting that Vas[16] found indirect evidence of testosterone deficiency in 66% of men with MS who reported complete lack of erection, and in 37% who reported partial erectile dysfunction. However, these men also had neurological symptoms which could as easily have explained their erectile problems. Such symptoms do not appear in Vas's research study. Indeed, even if future work confirms the finding of testosterone deficiency in men with MS (Vas acknowledged the limitations of his methodology), the reduced hormone levels could have been the result of diminished sexual activity rather than the cause of erectile dysfunction.[41]

Fertility and Contraception

While it has been reported that MS symptoms may vary during the menstrual cycle,[42] I have seen no reports on reduced fertility in women as a result of MS. Although contradictory opinions exist concerning the effects of pregnancy on the condition,[20,43,44] the possibility of becoming pregnant is apparently unaffected.

Are any of the commonly used contraceptive methods contraindicated for women with MS? It has been reported that birth control pills may aggravate the symptoms of MS;[45] but Burnfield[20] says she has been unable to find the evidence to document this claim (i.e. that the 'pill' holds unique risks for women with MS beyond those for the general population). She would prescribe the 'pill' for a woman with MS but would monitor her carefully for the first few months.

The IUD might be contraindicated if adductor spasms of the thighs or other disabilities create problems with menstrual hygiene,[20] and also in the case of reduced abdominal sensation, since warning of side-effects (e.g. pelvic pains or cramps) might be less noticeable.[38] Barrier methods that require some manual dexterity for effective use may be impractical in the presence of severe disability; but in mild cases it appears that any effective method would be appropriate.[20]

Sperm production is probably unaffected in men with MS; but the ability to obtain an erection or to ejaculate may be altered and this may, in turn, reduce the chances of a man with MS impregnating his partner. Under these circumstances it may be possible to collect motile spermatozoa by electrically stimulating the ejaculatory reflex and then using the sperm for artificial insemination. This technique has been used with spinal-cord-injured men and experiments are currently underway to improve the procedure.[46]

Condom use by a man with MS would be impractical only in cases of disability that altered manual dexterity, and even this is not necessarily a disadvantage unless his partner is similarly disabled. Condoms give the added advantage of protection against venereal disease, minimal side-effects and male involvement in contraception, a responsibility often carried disproportionately by women. Surgical sterilisation for either male or female is another highly reliable method of contraception for those who do not wish for more (or any) children. It is currently the most commonly used method in the world and, to my knowledge, carries no MS-related side-effects or contraindications.

A number of important sexual side-effects can accompany MS either as a direct result of neurological damage or as an indirect effect of the disease, or both. These effects can occur even in the absence of severe disability and can alter the frequency, type and enjoyment of sexual activity.

However, MS does not and should not spell an end to sexual pleasure and satisfaction. Knowledge of the sexual implications of the disease, coupled with a willingness to experiment and to communicate openly about them can help people to cope with changes in their sexual responses and relationships. Counsellors who share this information and encourage discussion about sexual concerns can defuse minor problems before they develop into larger, relationship-threatening crises.

REFERENCES

1. Smith B. H. (1976). Multiple sclerosis and sexual dysfunction. *Medical Aspects of Human Sexuality*; **10**:103.
2. Lundberg P.O. (1978). Sexual dysfunction in patients with multiple sclerosis. *Sexuality and Disability*. **1**:218.
3. Masters W.H., Johnson V.E. (1966). *Human Sexual Response*. Boston: Little, Brown.

4. Comarr A.E. (1971). Sexual concepts in traumatic cord and cauda equiva lesions. *Journal of Urology*; **106**:375.
5. Comarr A.E. (1978). Sex classification and expectations among quadriplegics and paraplegics. *Sexuality and Disability*; **1**:252.
6. Tarabulcy E. (1972). Sexual function in the normal and in paraplegia. *Paraplegia*; **10**:201.
7. Weiss H.D. (1972). The physiology of human penile erection. *Annals of Internal Medicine*; **76**:793.
8. Horenštein S. (1976) Sexual dysfunction in neurological disease. *Medical Aspects of Human Sexuality*; **10**:6.
9. Geiger R. (1977). Sexual implications of spinal cord injury. In *Physical Medicine and Rehabilitation Approaches in Spinal Cord Injury* (Cull J., Hardy R., eds.) pp. 54–86. Illinois: Charles C Thomas.
10. Geiger R.C. (1979). Neurophysiology of sexual response in spinal cord injury. *Sexuality and Disability*; **2**:257.
11. Money J. (1960). Phantom orgasm in the dreams of paraplegic men and women. *Archives of General Psychology*; **3**:373.
12. Higgins G.E. (1979). Sexual response in spinal cord injured adults: A review of the literature. *Archives of Sexual Behaviour*; **8**:173.
13. Cohen H.D., Rosen R.C., Goldstein L. (1976). Electroencephalographic laterality changes during human sexual orgasm. *Archives of Sexual Behaviour*; **5**:189.
14. Bregman S. (1978). Sexual adjustment of spinal cord injured women. *Sexuality and Disability*; **1**:85.
15. Ivers R.R., Goldstein N.P. (1963). Multiple sclerosis: A current appraisal of symptoms and signs. *Proceedings of the Mayo Clinic*; **38**:457.
16. Vas C.J. (1969). Sexual impotence and some autonomic disturbances in men with multiple sclerosis. *Acta Neurologica Scandinavica*; **45**:166.
17. Julty S. (1979). *Men's Bodies, Men's Selves*. Dell.
18. Lilius H.G., Valtonen E.J., Wikström J. (1976). Sexual problems in patients suffering from multiple sclerosis. *Journal of Chronic Diseases*; **29**:643.
19. Schneider E. (1974). Storungen der Sexualfunktion bei Nichttraumatischen Ruckenmarkerserkrankungen. *Fortschr. Neuro-Psychiat*; **42**:562.
20. Burnfield P. (1978). Sexual problems and multiple sclerosis. *British Journal of Family Planning*; **4**:2.
21. Miller H, Simpson C.A., Yeates W.K. (1965). Bladder dysfunction in multiple sclerosis. *British Medical Journal*; **1**:1265.
22. Pulton T.W. (1975). Multiple sclerosis: experience of personal alienation. *The Canadian Nurse*: July 16–18.
23. Carrera M.A., Kelley S. (1979). The right to a sexual life. *MS Quarterly*; **2**:4.
24. Barrett F.M. (1981). *Sexuality and Multiple Sclerosis*. Toronto: Multiple Sclerosis Society of Canada.
25. Lundberg P.O. (1977). Neurological examination of patients with sexual dysfunction. *Medical Aspects of Human Sexuality*; **11**:59.
26. Pearman R.O. (1972). Insertion of a Silastic penile prosthesis for the treatment of organic sexual impotence. *Journal of Urology*; **107**:802.

27. Scott F.B., Bradley W.E., Timm G.W. (1973). Erectile impotence. *Urology*; **2**:80.
28. Small M.P., Carrion H.M., Gordon J.A. (1975) Small-Carrion penile prosthesis. *Urology*; **5**:479.
29. Furlow W.L. (1978). Surgical treatment of impotence using the inflatable penile prosthesis. *Sexuality and Disability*; **1**:299.
30. Lange P.H., Smith A.D. (1978). A comparison of the two types of penile prosthesis used in the surgical treatment of male impotence. *Sexuality and Disability*; **1**:299.
31. Melman A. (1978). Erectile impotence. *Sexuality and Disability*; **1**:272.
32. Karacan I., Ilaria R.L. (1978). Nocturnal penile tumescence (NPT): The phenomenon and its role in the diagnosis of impotence. *Sexuality and Disability*; **1**:260.
33. Maddock J.W. (1980). Assessment and evaluation protocol for surgical treatment of impotence. *Sexuality and Disability*; **3**:39.
34. Marshall P., Surridge D., Delva N. (1981). The role of nocturnal penile tumescence in differentiating between organic and psychogenic impotence: The first stage of validation. *Archives of Sexual Behaviour*; **10**:1.
35. Bullard D.G., Mann J., Caplan H., Stoklosa J.M. (1978). Sex counseling and the penile prosthesis. *Sexuality and Disability*; **1**:184.
36. Small M.P. (1978). The Small-Carrion penile prosthesis: surgical implant for the management of impotence. *Sexuality and Disability*; **1**:282.
37. Rabin B. (1980). *The Sensuous Wheeler: Sexual Adjustment for the Spinal Cord Injured*. San Francisco: Multi Media Resource Center.
38. Shaul, S., Bogle J., Jale-Harbaugh J., Norman A.D. (1978). *Family Planning and Sexuality Concerning Physically Disabled Women*. New York: Human Sciences Press.
39. Zuckerman M. (1971). Physiological measures of sexual arousal in the human. *Psychological Bulletin*; **75**:297.
40. Herold E., Mottin J., Sabry Z. (1979). Effect of vitamin E on human sexual functioning. *Archives of Sexual Behaviour*; **8**:397.
41. Kraemer H.C., Becker H.B., Brodie H.K.H., Doering C.H., Moos R.H., Hamburg D.A. (1976). Orgasmic frequency and plasma testosterone levels in normal human males. *Archives of Sexual Behaviour*; **5**:125.
42. McAlpine D., Lumsden C.E., Acheson E.D. (1972). *Multiple Sclerosis: A Reappraisal*. London: Churchill Livingstone.
43. Humbert L.R., Carpenter R.J., O'Grady J.W. (1953). Pregnancy associated with mutliple sclerosis. *American Journal of Obstetrics and Gynecology*; **66**:403.
44. Cohen H.R., Krueger H.G. (1955). Multiple sclerosis and pregnancy. *Obstetrics and Gynecology*; **6**:144.
45. Heslinga K., Schellen A.M.C.M., Verkuyl A. (1974). *Not Made of Stone—The Sexual Problems of Handicapped People*. Illinois: Charles C Thomas.
46. Brindley G.S. (1980). Electroejaculation and fertility of paraplegic men. *Sexuality and Disability*; **3**:223.

Emotional Disorder in Multiple Sclerosis

At the time of writing this chapter Tony Whitlock was Professor of Psychiatry at the University of Queensland, Australia, with special interest in MS.

In this chapter he considers the relationship of emotional symptoms to the disease process in MS. He discusses the depression developed by many people with MS as a reaction to their illness (as well as the state of euphoria often encountered) and distinguishes this from the endogenous depression and mania resulting from cerebral damage— which may be an early sign of the disease.

The treatment appropriate for such emotional disorders and its efficacy are reviewed and numerous references are given for those interested in looking further into the subject.

Although cognitive impairment has long been recognised as one of the complications of MS, the precise relationship of affective (emotional) symptoms to the disease process is less certain. In this respect, the paper by Cottrell and Wilson[1] has had a profound influence on what has been taught about the kind of changes to be expected in patients with MS. They reported that 63% of their patients showed an inappropriate degree of euphoria; whereas only 10% were depressed. In all, 84% expressed a feeling of physical well-being, even in the presence of advanced or severe neurological impairment; while 97% of the patients showed emotional lability.

An unjustified state of optimism and loss of emotional control were considered by the authors to be direct consequences of the disease process and not psychogenic in origin. They claimed that they had specifically excluded intellectual deterioration as the likely cause as this was observed in only 2 of their 100 patients. As a consequence, an inappropriate euphoria has for many decades been regarded as one of the cardinal symptoms of MS, in conjunction with Charcot's triad of nystagmus, intention tremor and dysarthria.

This opinion is contrary to Runge's[2], who considered that euphoria was the result of the intellectual deterioration observed, usually, in the later stages of the disease; whereas depression was common during the earlier stages. Today, Runge's views are more generaly accepted;[3-6] but no satisfactory explanation for the discordant findings of Cottrell and Wilson has ever been given. In contrast to their observation that 63% of their patients were euphoric, later observers have found evidence for this in far fewer cases. Braceland and Giffin[3] considered that only 10% of their patients were euphoric, in contrast with 20% who were depressed. Surridge[6] found that 26% of his patients were euphoric, but a further 27% were depressed. In a study of patients in Israel, euphoria was recorded in only 5% and depression in 6% of patients; 3% of whom committed suicide, a rate that was some 14 times greater than in the general Israel population. Pratt[5] commented more particularly on emotional lability (35%) but only 6% of his patients admitted to a sense of increased physical well-being. It is important to distinguish between the outward manifestations of mood and the patient's true inner feelings, lest an apparent labile cheerfulness be taken to represent a far different affective state.[8] Surridge found that 8 of 28 euphoric patients were in fact feeling depressed. He considered that euphoria, which was associated with intellectual deterioration in all but two examples, was a pathological phenomenon, the direct result of damage to the central nervous system.

DEPRESSION

On common-sense grounds, it might be expected that patients with a progressively incapacitating disease with repeated remissions and relapses would be depressed. The belief that depression is an understandable response to the illness is held by a number of writers.[6,9,10,11] Lishman[12] states: 'Depression appears to be reactive in origin in the majority of cases and there is little reason to suspect that it is founded in cerebral pathology'. Surridge similarly asserts that 'depressive states occur in multiple sclerosis with far greater frequency than has been considered hitherto' and that 'they are psychogenic or reactive in nature'. Lurati *et al.*,[11] on the other hand, found that the depth of depression was associated with increasing severity of neurological symptoms: a finding which suggests that in some patients at least cerebral damage could have been a possible cause. Similarly, Braceland and Giffin[3] observed both euphoria and depression in patients with evidence of organic deterioration. Consequently, one might argue that in some patients depression is as likely as euphoria to be the result of brain damage, and that the former response is no more a psychogenic reaction than the inappropriate euphoria. In short, there is evidence that in some cases, manic–depressive or purely depressive symptoms will occur as a result of brain damage. Indeed, one would hardly expect otherwise in the face of evidence that physical disease directly or indirectly affecting the brain will sometimes be associated with severe depression or mania.[13,14] Nonetheless, observations of this kind pose a number of problems requiring solution before one can say with any firm assurance that an affective disorder is being caused directly and solely by the underlying brain lesion.

1. When depression occurs in the setting of physical disease, is the patient suffering from depression as a *symptom* or a *syndrome*? When patients become depressed without the associated physical and psychological features of an endogenous mood change, it seems reasonable to regard the symptom as a response to adversity, a kind of grief reaction which in purely human terms is readily comprehensible. On the other hand, some patients develop the characteristic symptoms and signs of the depressive phase of manic–depressive psychosis; and others may become manic, a syndrome which is far less likely to be a simple reaction to misfortune.

2. In patients with MS who develop a picture of endogenous depression, to what extent can one determine whether this is an illness which has been released by the disease in a predisposed subject? The presence of a positive family history of affective disorder or a past personal history of such illness long before neurological signs and symptoms appear might suggest that severe depression, once the diagnosis of MS is established, has come about as a release phenomenon which could have occurred as a result of any number of cerebral insults. In some of these patients, the mood changes might also be precipitated by medication, particularly steroids.

3. On the other hand, there are patients with neither positive family histories nor past personal histories of affective disorder who develop severe depression shortly before the appearance of neurological symptoms of MS, or who become psychiatrically ill some time after the transient appearance of neurological symptoms which only retrospectively are diagnosed correctly. Possibly the best account of severe depression as a presenting symptom of MS was provided by Barbellion in *The Journal of a Disappointed Man*.[15] He described the sudden descent of severe melancholia when, as he put it, 'all the colour went out of my life and the world was dirty grey'. At times he was troubled by suicidal thoughts and it is worth recording, as Pratt has done,[5] how Barbellion was well aware of the disparity between his outward appearance of normality or gaiety and his inner feelings of clouded depression and foreboding.

Reports of depression before neurological symptoms appear have been made by a number of authors. For example, six cases of MS have been described which started with depression whose causes were only diagnosed when neurological signs suddenly appeared.[16] Similarly, it has been recorded that psychiatric illness sometimes precedes the onset of physical symptoms:[17] the three patients examined all showed evidence of dementia and one was depressed. An important example was provided by Bignami *et al.*[18] who described the onset of severe depression in a 22-year-old man one month before symptoms of neurological disease appeared. There was no past history of depression in this patient, who deteriorated rapidly and died. At autopsy he was found to have plaques of demyelination in the hypothalamus, cerebral peduncles and pons. The hypothalamic lesions were thought to be responsible for his severe mood changes and one might, on anatomical grounds, assume that in other patients lesions in various parts of the limbic brain would cause affective changes of sufficient severity to justify a diagnosis of endogenous depression or mania.

Young *et al.*[19] considered that mental changes can be early features of MS before physical signs of the disease appear. Two of their five patients were depressed and successfully treated. These authors related the affective symptoms to brainstem lesions and widespread cerebral demyelination, and considered that the frequency of early psychiatric symptoms in MS has been underestimated. Crémieux *et al.*[20] described a 47-year-old man who for a year had suffered from neurological symptoms of moderate severity, but who developed a manic–depressive psychosis. There was no past history or family history of affective disorder. At autopsy, plaques of demyelination in both temporal lobes and the thalamus were regarded as the causes of his affective symptoms. A survey of 200 reports on MS found only 15 which mentioned emotional difficulties before the onset of physical symptoms.[21] Only 5 suggested a common pathogenic process for both physical and psychological symptoms. This apparent absence of interest in the psychological status of their patients on the part of neurologists is disconcerting but by no means unusual. For example, a monograph on MS based on 1062 patients seen by the authors[22] is quite remarkably uninformative about the mental states of the patients, some of whom are described in considerable neurological detail. Goodstein and Ferrell failed to find any paper in which depression was the presenting feature of MS, but went on to record it in three patients of their own. One of these, a 33-year-old woman, with diffuse cortical impairment and severe depressive illness of three months' duration, failed to respond to treatment. She had shown signs of remitting and relapsing neurological symptoms for some years before her present admission. In addition, she had suffered from recurrent psychiatric illnesses described as 'depression and nervousness'. O'Malley,[23] in his review of the older literature, was manifestly concerned at the relative lack of information on the mental state of MS patients, either before or after the onset of the disease. Charcot, an exception, commented on intellectual impairment, euphoria, depression and psychosis as occurring in some patients. Other writers emphasised 'hysteria' as a common feature of the condition and in some instances suicide is mentioned as the consequence of severe mental disorders. O'Malley described three patients with mental changes, one of whom, a 35-year-old man, suffered from two attacks of depression before the onset of MS symptoms. He had suicidal ideas during the second attack, from which he did not make a complete recovery. Ultimately he became demented and died. Plaques and demyelination were observed throughout the cerebral cortex and basal ganglia.

A 40-year-old female patient has been described who first developed neurological symptoms at the age of 25, with a recurrence at the age of 33.[24] Three years later she became severely depressed. Details have also been given of three patients with remitting psychoses preceding the onset of physical symptoms of MS.[25] Although diagnosed as schizophrenic, one might consider that the second patient was severely depressed. She recovered completely and later developed neurological signs of MS. Another example is that of a 61-year-old woman who was grossly psychotic and neglected in association with MS.[26] She had a past history of recurrent depression extending over a period of 36 years. Despite her severe psychosis, she responded well to lithium therapy and no longer manifested a state of severe degradation and self-neglect. In this patient, the later development of MS appears to have precipitated an affective disorder in someone predisposed to this reaction by earlier attacks of depression.

Although the papers so far mentioned have emphasised severe depression as the presenting feature of MS, it is evident that mania can also occur, as in the case described by Crémieux *et al.*[20] One patient became manic in association with predominantly brainstem signs of MS.[27] Another report is of a 35-year-old woman with a ten-year history of MS.[28] She became severely depressed and later manic in response to treatment with ACTH. Her past history of cyclothymia appears to have been the crucial factor determining her response to treatment, although conceivably her predisposition to mood change could have been caused by her neurological disease.

From these reports, it is clear that by no means all MS patients with severe affective disturbances are examples of reactive depression. In some cases, current depression of a typically endogenous kind has been experienced for some years before the onset of MS. In such cases, a recurrence of psychiatric symptoms in association with neurological disease could be regarded as coincidental. Alternatively, the psychosis may have been precipitated by brain damage in a predisposed patient. On the other hand, some patients develop severe affective disturbances shortly before the onset of neurological symptoms and in such cases it is likely that the psychiatric disorder was the presenting symptom of a disease process which had not yet manifested features characteristic of MS. Once the condition is established, it is very difficult to decide whether the depression is endogenous or reactive, and in all probability no single explanation will cover all cases. With some of these complexities in mind, a comparison was made of 30 patients suffering from MS with 30 matched control patients suffering from a variety of neurological disorders of a chronic disabling kind.[29]

The MS cases and controls were well matched for the degree of disability. All patients were assessed for evidence of past and present affective disorder and all completed the Beck Depressive Inventory. The MS patients scored significantly higher on this rating scale than the controls. Their scores correlated to some extent with the degree of disability being experienced. Fourteen of the MS patients were depressed at the time of the interview, compared with two controls. Eight of the MS patients had suffered from depression before the onset of neurological symptoms and two of these had experienced transitory neurological symptoms which had not been diagnosed at the time. Sixteen of the MS patients and five controls had episodes of endogenous depression since the onset of their neurological illnesses. Because patients who were showing clear signs of dementia were excluded, euphoria was not observed, but five showed marked fluctuation of mood with depression predominating. On the other hand, some of the patients did show evidence of cerebral or brainstem involvement characterised by impaired memory, epilepsy and severe dysarthria. At least one patient attempted suicide and others had contemplated taking their lives. One patient, not included in the series of 30, developed manic–depressive psychosis after the onset of MS and finally committed suicide in the depressive phase of his illness. Although many patients had been and were still receiving steroids and/or Baclofen, it did not appear that these drugs were contributing to their affective states. The following short case histories illustrate some of the features shown by these patients.

1. A woman aged 28 first developed neurological symptoms at the age of 23, with a recurrence three years later. At the age of 27 she became severely depressed with delusions of guilt and the belief that Satan was inhabiting her body. She made a serious suicidal attempt from which she

was resuscitated, but continued to be severely depressed and potentially suicidal.

2. A woman aged 52 first developed MS symptoms at the age 35. At the age of 51, she showed evidence of early organic deterioration and was severely depressed and suicidal. She died and at autopsy large plaques and demyelination were found, predominantly in the left temporal and parietal regions.

3. A woman aged 50 was first diagnosed as suffering from MS at the age of 42. By the age of 48 she was severely disabled and depressed and attempted suicide by drug overdose.

The symptoms and signs of affective disorder in most of these patients were characteristically those of the depressive phase of manic–depressive psychosis, confirmed by their responses on the Beck Inventory. Although a number of environmental factors could well have aggravated their symptoms, it could hardly be said that these patients were suffering from psychogenic reactive disorders. On the other hand, some patients who were manifestly depressed at the time of interview and scored highly on the Beck Depressive Inventory were more clearly examples of a neurotic depressive reaction.

TREATMENT

Apart from the general support, both social and psychotherapeutic, which is essential for the management of patients with MS, it is apparent that patients with severe affective disorders may need more specific treatment. A number of writers have observed how severe depression coming on in the course of MS or anteceding the onset of the disease responds well to tricyclic antidepressants or electroconvulsive therapy.[16, 17, 19] In this respect, these patients do not differ from others with depression following brain damage, and one might consider that this therapeutic response gives some support to the belief that affective changes can be precipitated by brain damage in the course of MS. Kemp *et al.*[28] used lithium to treat their cyclothymic patient suffering from MS and agitated depression. Later, in response to steroid treatment, she became manic. Another patient with MS and recurrent depression did not respond to tricyclic antidepressants but finally recovered with the administration of lithium.[26]

In contrast to these reports, none of the three patients described by Goodstein and Ferrell[21] responded to antidepressant treatment. It is interesting to note that Matthews' second patient, who appeared to be psychotic and depressed, finally settled with steroid treatment which also ameliorated her physical symptoms.[25] Earlier she had been treated with chlorpromazine without improvement.

Finally, the experience of sufferers from MS can provide valuable information showing how severe depression in the course of the illness can respond to tricyclic antidepressants.[30] Burnfield also emphasises the need to continue with counselling and intensive psychotherapy in conjunction with drugs or ECT.

In general, therefore, severe depression or manic–depressive psychosis occurring in the course of MS will often respond satisfactorily to appropriate treatment, despite the likely coexistence of brain damage. There is no place for therapeutic nihilism in the total management of both psychological and physical disabilities in patients with this disease.

In summary, it has been shown that although many patients with MS will develop depression as an understandable reaction to their illnesses, others more clearly suffer from endogenous depression which could be the direct consequence of cerebral damage. Pathological evidence implicates areas of the brain such as the frontal lobes and other parts of the limbic system whose impairment through disease or injury often results in serious depression or, less frequently, mania. The very widespread lesions in the brains of MS patients will almost certainly affect these areas whose functions are of prime importance for the experience and expression of emotion. In such cases, severe depression is an understandable development in the course of, or as the presenting syndrome of, a progressive neurological disease.

REFERENCES

1. Cottrell S.S., Wilson S.A.K. (1926). The affective symptomatology of disseminated sclerosis. *Journal of Neurology and Psychopathology*; **7**:1.
2. Runge W. (1928). In *Bumke's Handbuch der Geisteskrankheiten*; 7:616. (Quoted in Surridge, 1979).
3. Braceland F.J., Giffin M.E. (1950). The mental changes associated with multiple sclerosis (an interim report). *Association for Research in Nervous and Mental Diseases*, Vol. 28, pp. 450–55. Baltimore: Williams & Wilkins.
4. Canter A.H. (1951). Direct and indirect measures of psychological deficit in multiple sclerosis. *Journal of General Psychology*; **44**:3, 27.
5. Pratt R.T.C. (1951). An investigation of the psychiatric aspects of disseminated sclerosis. *Journal of Neurology, Neurosurgery and Psychiatry*; **14**:326.
6. Surridge D. (1969). An investigation into some psychiatric aspects of multiple sclerosis. *British Journal of Psychiatry*; **115**:749.

7. Kahana E., Leibowitz A., Alter M. (1971). Cerebral multiple sclerosis. *Neurology*; **21**:1179.
8. Burnfield A., Burnfield P. (1978). Common psychological problems in multiple sclerosis. *British Medical Journal*; **1**:1193.
9. Gaillinek A., Kalinowsky L.B. (1958). Psychiatric aspects of multiple sclerosis. *Diseases of the Nervous System*; **19**:77.
10. Kurtzke J.F. (1970) Clinical manifestations of multiple sclerosis. In *Handbook of Clinical Neurology*, Vol. 9 (Vinken P.J., Bruyn C.W., eds.) pp. 161–216. Amsterdam: North-Holland.
11. Lurati M., Bottenberg E.H., Lützenkirchen J., Schoefer M. (1976). Multiple Sklerose und Persönlichkeitsaspektre. *Archives für Psychiatrie und Nervenkrankheiten*; **221**:303.
12. Lishman W.A. (1978). *Organic Psychiatry*. Oxford: Blackwell Scientific.
13. Hendrie H.C. (1978). *Brain Disorders: Clinical Diagnosis and Management*. Psychiatric Clinics of North America, Vol. 1/1. Philadelphia: W.B. Saunders.
14. Krauthammer C., Klerman G.L. (1978). Secondary mania. *Archives of General Psychiatry*; **35**:1333.
15. Barbellion W.N.P. (1919). *The Journal of a Disappointed Man*. London: Chatto and Windus.
16. Pommé B., Girard J., Planche R. (1963). Forme dépressive de début d'ime sclérose en plaques. *Annales Medico-Psychologique*; **121**:133.
17. Mur J., Kümpel G., Dostál S. (1966). An anergic phase of disseminated sclerosis with psychiatric course. *Confina Neurologica*; **28**:37.
18. Bignami A., Gherardi D., Gallo G. (1961). Sclerosi a placche acuta a localizzazione i potalamica con sintomologia psychica di tipo malinconico. *Rivista di Neurologia*; **31**:240.
19. Young A.C., Saunders J., Ponsford J.R. (1976). Mental change as an early feature of multiple sclerosis. *Journal of Neurology, Neurosurgery and Psychiatry*; **39**:1008.
20. Crémieux A., Alliez J., Tonga M., Pache R. (1959). Sclérose en plaques a début par troubles mentaux: étude anatomo-clinique. *Révue Neurologique*; **101**:45.
21. Goodstein R.K., Ferrell R.B. (1977). Multiple sclerosis presenting as a depressive illness. *Diseases of the Nervous System*; **38**:127.
22. McAlpine D., Compston N.D., Lumsden C.E. (1955). *Multiple Sclerosis*. Edinburgh: E. & S. Livingstone.
23. O'Malley P.P. (1966). Severe mental symptoms in disseminated sclerosis: a neuropathological study. *Journal of the Irish Medical Association*; **58**:115.
24. Caplan L.R., Nadelson T. (1980). Multiple sclerosis and hysteria. *Journal of the American Medical Association*; **243**:2418.
25. Matthews W.B. (1979). Multiple sclerosis presenting with acute remitting psychiatric symptoms. *Journal of Neurology, Neurosurgery and Psychiatry*; **42**:859.
26. Mehta D.B. (1976). Lithium and affective disorders associated with organic brain impairment. *American Journal of Psychiatry*; **133**:236.

27. Targowla H. (1927). Sclérose en plaques fruste a début mental. *L'Encephale*; **22**:169. (Quoted in Matthews, 1979.)
28. Kemp K., Lion J.R., Magram G. (1977). Lithium in the treatment of a manic patient with multiple sclerosis: a case report. *Diseases of the Nervous System*; **38**:210.
29. Whitlock F.A., Siskind D.M.M. (1980). Depression as a major symptom of multiple sclerosis. *Journal of Neurology, Neurosurgery and Psychiatry*; **43**:861.
30. Burnfield A. (1977). Multiple sclerosis: a doctor's personal experience. *British Medical Journal*; **1**:435.

Neuropsychological Findings

Lindsay Vowels is the neuropsychologist with the Victorian Multiple Sclerosis Society in Australia, and Gerry Gates is Lecturer in Psychology with the University of Melbourne and is presently supervising Lindsay's PhD thesis on MS.

In this chapter they relate the psychological reactions discussed in the previous chapter to deterioration in the central nervous system that occurs as a result of MS. The chapter is based on a neuropsychological study carried out by the authors to assess the effects of frontal-lobe impairment on the performances of people with MS.

The authors stress the importance of being aware of the variability in the deterioration of skills in people with MS, and of the fact that intellectual and behavioural deterioration due to frontal-lobe damage may occur in some, while others remain mentally intact.

The results of the authors' study indicate that careful neuropsychological evaluation is important in order to tailor management programmes to individuals with MS.

A neuropsychological study of MS involves investigation of the neurological basis of intellectual and emotional changes accompanying the disease. These aspects of MS have received very little attention compared to the diversity of studies which have probed the aetiology and physical pathology of the problem. Changes in intellectual performance and personality function have been reported in MS patients for at least 100 years: psychomotor impairment, memory deterioration, depression and euphoria have been among the most frequent problems noted. Many of these changes have been regarded as psychological reactions to the effects of physical disability or to alteration in social circumstances as a result of the disease, or as an affective response to having an incurable illness.

Little attention has been paid to the possible role that actual deterioration in the central nervous system might play in psychological changes accompanying the disease. Although many of the cognitive and behavioural abnormalities which have been reported as 'common' in MS resemble the changes which occur with lesions in the frontal lobes, no study has examined the possible association of psychological changes in MS patients and organic impairment of the frontal regions.

An investigation (carried out by the authors) of frontal-lobe function in a group of 100 MS patients using neuropsychological tests sensitive to frontal-lobe impairment revealed deficits in the performance of MS patients when compared to that of a matched control group.

Deficits observed in MS patients were only poorly correlated with duration of illness, age of patient, and severity of physical disability. The study suggested that the alteration of cognitive abilities and affective function in the MS group is due to organic deterioration of the frontal lobes as a result of the disease process, rather than to affective reaction to the disease. Frontal-lobe impairment may be a more frequent problem in MS than has been recognised previously, and may contribute significantly to the substantial problems of adjustment, new learning and rehabilitation experienced by many MS patients.

The earliest descriptions of the psychological characteristics of MS reveal that changes in mental function were a common feature of the disease. In his treatise on MS, Charcot noted 'There is marked enfeeblement of the memory: conceptions are formed slowly: the intellectual and emotional faculties are blunted in their totality'.[1]

Recent investigations of the psychological features of MS have examined a wide range of functions, and various reports suggest that some degree of psychological disturbance is common in the disease well before patients reach an advanced state.[2,3]

Many clinicians have commented on the reduced insight and poor adjustment shown by MS patients.[4,5] That some patients do not benefit from rehabilitation or retraining programmes[5,6] has been ascribed to lack of motivation or inconsistent application to the task at hand.[7] While many of the changes in behaviour and intellect in MS, such as poor motivation, irritability, poor concentration, lack of insight, perseverative behaviour, euphoria, and poor planning,[8] seem to have no common causal explanation, such changes are frequently associated with frontal-lobe impairment.[9–12]

The cerebral demyelination and plaque formation of MS, especially in the frontal lobes of MS patients, may be at least partially responsible for many of the intellectual, affective, and behavioural disturbances found in MS patients. It may help to explain, for example, behavioural difficulties as diverse as inability to track a moving target properly,[13] or euphoria.[8]

'Frontal-lobe syndrome' describes a variety of intellectual deficits, personality changes and behavioural abnormalities found in patients with lesions of the frontal lobes and has been described by many neuropsychologists.[10,11] Intellectual changes are characterised by impairment in memory and ability for new learning, decline of the capacity to plan and organise, reduction in flexibility of thinking and attitude, and deterioration in the ability to analyse and solve problems. Personality changes and behavioural abnormalities may include impairment of self-control, concentration and arousal; emotional lability; lack of insight and self-evaluation; increase in perseveration; rigidity of attitude and insensitivity to the needs and viewpoints of others; failure to benefit by experience; and inability to adapt to new situations.

The severity of each deficit varies considerably, depending on the site and extent of the underlying pathology, the age and premorbid status of the individual, and the conditions under which the behaviours are observed.[12]

Patients with frontal-lobe syndrome gain minimal benefit from prolonged rehabilitation. They experience difficulty in obtaining permanent employment and in establishing and maintaining ongoing relationships with others, irrespective of any additional physical disability they may also have. Such problem patients are commonly reported in the MS literature and amongst the helping professionals who work in the field.[3,14,15]

Neuropathological studies of MS do not emphasise the extent and frequency of demyelination found in the frontal lobes, but most neuroanatomic studies report that demyelination and plaque formation are frequently seen in the white matter of the periventricular regions and the corpus callosum.[16-19]

The periventricular regions surrounding the anterior horn of the lateral ventricles and the anterior aspects of the third ventricle are among the sites of demyelinating lesions in many MS cases.[18] Lesions in these areas may have interruptive effects on a number of important associative tracts connecting the frontal cortex with the basal ganglia and other cortical and subcortical areas. Neuropsychological evidence suggests that disruption to these tracts results in significant impairment of cognitive functions in the manner of other 'disconnection' lesions.[10] In the case of MS patients, the frontal lobes could be functionally disconnected, leaving the rest of the brain without the superordinate, master control of the frontal lobes, the importance of which has been stressed by Walsh.[11]

The literature concerning the psychological effects of MS has not considered frontal-lobe damage as a possible explanation for the diverse changes in both emotional and cognitive capacity in MS patients;[7,8,20-23] although Pratt[1] has suggested that the disappearance of long-standing psychiatric problems in MS patients may reflect interruption of the frontothalamic tracts by plaque formation which 'might produce an anatomical and functional change similar to that following pre-frontal leucotomy'. However, this lack of emphasis on a frontal-lobe explanation may reflect the fact that earlier studies did not use psychological tests and observation measures which were sufficiently sensitive to detect the subtle alterations in function which may occur with disruption to the frontal-lobe tracts, and did not recognise the diverse behavioural and intellectual changes as possibly reflecting a single causal entity.

A study by the authors examined emotional and intellectual changes in MS patients using neuropsychological measures which tap frontal-lobe function. This study found that when compared to a normal control group, a group of MS patients showed significant intellectual deficits over time. The incidence of cognitive impairment was higher than previous estimates which describe significant intellectual deterioration only as a late or terminal feature of the disease.[23-25] Unrepresentative or small samples in other studies and inadequate or insensitive testing may account for much of the discrepancy among studies. Only when the results of the current (1982) epidemiological study of MS in Australia become available, will it be clear how representative of the MS population the sample of the authors' study was.

One important difference between this and previous studies was that the authors' study investigated intellectual impairment using tasks known to tap frontal-lobe function. It showed that MS patients do not exhibit uniform deterioration of intellect as in dementia, but rather undergo a selective reduction in certain abilities with relative sparing of others. The pattern of cognitive impairment includes at least three components: (1) serious deficits in 'dynamic' cognitive frontal functioning, such as ability to organise, plan, and problem-solve in a variety of unfamiliar situations; (2) moderate deterioration of memory and learning processes; and (3) preservation of automatic, long-standing and well-practised verbal skills.

An interesting finding was that only those who scored high on the continuum of intelligence also showed significant affective disturbance. Given the nature of the disease and the relatively poor prognosis for most patients, one would expect depression to be a common problem. The fact that objective signs of depression are mostly confined to those who are intellectually intact suggests that those who are impaired may have been protected from depression. Lack of insight resulting from disease in the frontal lobes, rather than acceptance of the disease state, may explain the low depression scores of the intellectually impaired patients. This lack of insight may develop as organic deterioration occurs and as consequent immobility progresses. This psychological change may be a 'blessing in disguise' for the patient, while making day-to-day management of that person extremely difficult.

As mentioned above, three main cognitive deficits are apparent in the scores of the MS patients investigated here. Of these deficits, memory impairment is the most common. It was the experience of one of the authors, in the testing of over 300 MS patients, that some degree of memory impairment is common, and may be an early diagnostic feature of the disease, rather than a late or end-stage characteristic of the disorder.

The second most common cognitive problem seen in the MS group relates to frontal-lobe impairment. Almost one-third of the MS patients displayed a marked deficit in all tests requiring planning, organisation, utilisation of feedback, and problem-solving. These patients also showed significant memory impairment and flattening of affect. In addition to this group, almost one-half of the patients showed signs of moderate impairment in the same tests, although only half of these patients had memory problems and/or flattening of affective reaction.

The third problem observed in the MS group was that of psychomotor impairment on all tests of performance requiring speed and fine motor co-ordination. The relative contribution of poor motor capacity to poor test performance is difficult to judge; however, because other non-neurological disabled control groups have performed on similar tests (see, for example, Vowels[26]) very much like the normal control group, poor motor capacity itself may not be a major contributor to many of the deficits observed in MS patients. The fact that MS patients do poorly on tests of frontal-lobe function not requiring skilful manipulation would suggest that motor deficit is not as important a determinant of poor test performance as the literature implies,[22] although its influence cannot be completely ruled out.

One shortcoming of the authors' study was that there was no anatomical evidence of lesions or plaques in the frontal lobes of the patients to substantiate the claim that poor performance on tests known to be sensitive to frontal function actually is correlated with frontal lesions. MS plaques are notoriously difficult to detect using current radiological techniques, and confirmation of neuropathology is certain only at autopsy.[18]

The group performance of MS patients deteriorated for all neuropsychological and most psychometric tests over three testing periods. Such deterioration was not seen in control subjects, who, in fact, exhibited some improvement in scores. The most marked deterioration for MS patients was in tests requiring memory, new learning and problem-solving ability, whereas little change was shown for verbal skills.

The practical implications of this fairly rapid and differential deterioration of cognitive skills are substantial. The MS population would appear to contain a significant number of individuals who are unable to or have difficulty in learning new skills, and in benefitting from training. They tend to make the same errors over and over again, and to forget material previously learned. This deterioration occurs at a time when they are also experiencing changes in their physical status, such as loss of muscle power and bladder function, as well as a change in body image and life-style. Many of these changes require some new learning: a new splint, a new pattern of compensatory walking, a new 'day programme' to attend, a new household to adapt to. Although these changes are usually carefully tailored to the physical 'needs' of the person, frequently no account is taken of the new learning requirements of the change. If an MS patient has frontal-lobe impairment, he may have great difficulty adapting to the new situation. Moreover, the intransigent behaviour of a patient having difficulty in learning may be interpreted by the therapist or teacher as stubborness or inflexibility. Such an impression is reinforced if the patient has reasonably intact verbal skills, and is able to repeat the rules or instructions of the task while being unable to carry them out.

In addition to the objective measures of frontal impairment as used in the study, a number of behavioural changes have also been observed which resemble those seen in frontal-lobe syndrome patients such as lack of insight, tendency to be impulsive or lowering of the level of arousal. Each of these behavioural alterations, in addition to other deficits exhibited by MS patients, may be extremely handicapping both to the MS patient and to those who are caring for him, and may make successful rehabilitation and management programmes very difficult.

Frontal-lobe deterioration may affect many aspects of the patient's life, including interpersonal relationships with others.[15] It is important that those who work and live with MS patients realise that many of the behavioural problems seen may reflect an organic problem, rather than the fact that the patient is just being purposely intractable or difficult to get along with. The erroneous assumption that MS affects only physical functions, but spares personality and cognitive abilities, is a view publicised by the popular press and some of the scientific literature.[23] Therefore, family members and hospital staff may blame the MS sufferer himself for unco-operative or selfish behaviour, rather than attributing such behaviours to the underlying organic cause. There is good evidence that both patients and family may benefit from being given information about the disease, no matter how discouraging that information may be.[5, 8, 27] It is important, though, that the extent of organic deterioration be determined objectively so that every difficulty encountered by the professional in assisting the patient is not attributed falsely to organic impairment. Moreover, testing may help the patient to understand his problems and avoid using organic impairment as an excuse for not doing things of which he is quite capable.

In view of the fact that frontal-lobe impairment is often accompanied by lack of insight, the question arises as to the effectiveness of initiating 'insightful' forms of psychotherapy or counselling with patients who exhibit objective signs of frontal damage. For those who are cognitively intact, such psychotherapy may be quite effective; but for those with flattened affect as a result of the disease, insightful psychotherapy may be inappropriate.

Another important aspect of the study described here was the finding that MS patients do not comprise a uniform group of individuals with the same problems. Intellectual deterioration was not seen in all patients and examination of the relationship between age, severity of physical disability and duration of illness showed that these factors were not good predictors of cognitive impairment. In view of the wide range of disabilities shown by patients and differences in mode of expression of the disease, some consideration should be given to the view that MS neuroanatomic evidence suggests that there are different forms of the disease.[28] Moreover, multiviral causes have been proposed and may explain these differences.[2]

The study also showed that a very substantial percentage of MS patients show signs of intellectual and behavioural deterioration consistent with damage to the frontal lobes. On the other hand, some MS patients may remain mentally intact, and although showing signs of depression or anxiety, are at least cognitively more amenable to effective individual rehabilitation programmes.

Careful neuropsychological evaluation is therefore essential to tailor a special programme of management to fit each individual.

ACKNOWLEDGEMENTS

The authors wish to thank Dr Anne Gates and Dr Peter Colville for their critical review of the manuscript. This research was supported, in part, by a Grant from the National Multiple Sclerosis Society of Australia Research Advisory Board.

EDITOR'S NOTE

The findings of Vowels' and Gates' study are important as objective evidence for their proposed theory that many psychological problems in

MS are in fact part of the disease process rather than reaction to it. For those interested in the way the investigation was carried out, contact with the authors at the Victorian Multiple Sclerosis Society, 616 Riversdale Road, Camberwell, Victoria, Australia, is recommended as this study was tightly controlled using the WAIS, NHAIS, Wechsler Memory Scale, The Austin Maze, the Goldstein Scheerer Colour Form Sorting Test, The Wisconsin Card Sorting Test, Halstead Category Test, Verbal Fluency Test and the MMPI.

REFERENCES

1. Pratt R.T.C. (1951). An investigation of the psychiatric aspects of disseminated sclerosis. *Journal of Neurology, Neurosurgery and Psychiatry*; **14**:326.
2. Ashworth B. (1980). The early diagnosis of multiple sclerosis. *Scottish Medical Journal*; **25**:58.
3. Peyser J.M., Edwards K.R., Poser M.D., Filskov S.R. (1980). Cognitive function in patients with multiple sclerosis. *Archives of Neurology*; **37**:577.
4. Bourestom N.S., Howard M.T. (1965). Personality characteristics of three disability groups. *Archives of Physiology, Medicine and Rehabilitation;* **46**:626.
5. Sedal L. (1980). Management of multiple sclerosis. *Patient Management*; **4**:69.
6. Liversedge L.A. (1977). Treatment and management of multiple sclerosis. *British Medical Bulletin*; **33**(1):78.
7. Schneitzer L. (1978). Rehabilitation of patients with multiple sclerosis. *Archives of Physiology, Medicine and Rehabilitation*; **59**:430.
8. Burnfield A., Burnfield P. (1978). Common psychological problems in multiple sclerosis. *British Medical Journal*; **1**:1193.
9. Benton A.L. (1968). Differential behaviour effects of frontal lobe disease. *Neuropsychologia*; **6**:53.
10. Luria A.R. (1973). *The Working Brain*. Harmondsworth: Penguin.
11. Walsh K.W. (1978). *Neuropsychology a Clinical Approach*. Edinburgh: Churchill Livingstone.
12. Damasio A. (1979). The frontal lobes.
In *The Frontal Lobes in Clinical Neuropsychology* (Heilman K.M., Valenstein E., eds.) pp. 370–421. New York: Oxford University Press.
13. Mastaglia F.L., Black J.L., Collins D.W.D. (1979). Quantitative studies of saccadic and pursuit eye movements in multiple sclerosis. *Brain*; **102**:817.
14. Miles A. (1979). Some psychosocial consequences of multiple sclerosis: problems of social interaction and group identity. *British Journal of Medical Psychology*; **52**:321.
15. Poser S., Raun N.E., Wikstrom J., Poser W. (1979). Pregnancy, oral contraceptives and multiple sclerosis. *Acta Neurologica Scandinavica*; **59**:108.

16. Barnard R.O., Triggs M. (1974). Corpus callosum in MS. *Journal of Neurology, Neurosurgery and Psychiatry*; **37**:1259.
17. Ikuta F., Zimmerman H.M. (1976). Distribution of plaques in seventy autopsy cases of multiple sclerosis in the United States. *Neurology (Minneapolis);* **26** (6 Pt 2):18.
18. Mastaglia F.L., Cala L.A. (1980). Computed tomography of the brain in MS. *Trends in Neurosciences*; **3**:16.
19. Morariu M.A., Wilkins D.E., Patel S. (1980). Multiple sclerosis and serial computerized tomography. *Archives of Neurology*; **37**:189.
20. Surridge D. (1969). An investigation into some psychiatric aspects of multiple sclerosis. *British Journal of Psychiatry*; **115**:749.
21. Weinstein E.A. (1970). Behavioural aspects of multiple sclerosis. *Modern Treatments*; **7**(5):961.
22. Beatty P.A., Gange J.J. (1977). Neuropsychological aspects of multiple sclerosis. *Journal of Nervous and Mental Diseases*; **164**(1):42.
23. Ivnik R.J. (1978). Neuropsychological test performance as a function of MS-related symptomatology. *Journal of Clinical Psychiatry*; **4**:304.
24. Canter A. (1951). Direct and indirect measures of psychological deficit in MS. *Journal of General Psychology;* **44**:3.
25. Reitan R.M., Reed J.C., Dyken M.L. (1971). Cognitive, psychomotor and motor correlates of multiple sclerosis. *Journal of Nervous and Mental Diseases*; **153**(3):218.
26. Vowels L.M. (1979). Memory impairment in multiple sclerosis. In *Brain Impairment: Proceedings of the Third Brain Impairment Workshop* (Molloy M., Stanley G.V., eds.) pp. 10–22. Parkville: Melbourne University Press.
27. Power P.W., Sax D.S. (1978). The communication of information to the neurological patient: some implications for family coping. *Journal of Chronic Diseases*; **31**:57.
28. Oppenheimer D.R. (1976). Demyelinating disease. In *Greenfield's Neuropathology* (Blackwood W., Corsellis J.A.N., eds.) pp. 470–99. Baltimore: Williams & Wilkins.

Society's Reaction to the Disabled: a Problem of Accessibility

In this chapter, Aart Simons discusses the attitudes of both the disabled and non-disabled towards disability— particularly the disability resulting from MS.

He examines the reasons for and forms of such prejudices and stigmatisation as are encountered — and their effects on the disabled and non-disabled — and suggests ways in which society's negative attitude towards disability can be overcome.

In addition to having to come face to face with realistic physical limitations imposed on them by their condition, MS-disabled people are forced to alter their self-concept as well— largely because of society's reaction to disability in general.

Western society, for example, places positive value on possessing an occupation, being productive at a job and achieving in the labour force.[1] Also highly valued are social interaction,[2] physical and emotional independence, physical attractiveness and youth,[3] as well as intact marriages, a cohesive family, children and active sexual lives.[4]

Physically disabled people frequently deviate from these norms and are therefore often regarded by themselves (due to the socialisation process) and others as less than normal: forming a group on its own.[5]

A truly modern society should perhaps be one that offers as many options as possible to all individuals, regardless of age, sex, social class, racial or ethnic origin or conditions of health; a society in which this range of options should be equally socially acceptable and desirable; a society in which people should be socialised to be totally free to take any of these options without later having to pay a social or psychological price; ideally, a society in which the disabled can be regarded as different, but equally acceptable to all.

However, a large gap exists between such an acceptable 'ideal' state and that of reality in most countries.

The status of disabled people has in fact varied throughout history and from country to country. Reaction to disability has ranged from complete rejection and ostracism to semi-deification and the giving of special privileges.[1]

In developing countries, particularly where medical facilities are scarce and large numbers of able-bodied persons are unemployed, the disabled are frequently totally rejected socially. Also, unless they have inherited wealth or are taken care of by their families, the disabled are reduced to begging.

In the more developed and Western societies, begging has virtually been eliminated and care for the disabled has been established through taxation and charity. However, a number of conditions remain which place the disabled, as a group, distinctly separate from the majority of society.[6] Modern society, in fact, tends to build upon a myth of an ideal society consisting of selected and approved individuals, of 'normal' human beings, with average intelligence, average bodily health and with a sufficient degree of maturity. These selected and privileged individuals feel they have to take care of the others who do not belong to this class of the 'true' society. This kind of care does not acknowledge the sick as belonging to the body unless they recover. In fact one might say that sick people do not belong to the true society. The prevalence of this idea is obvious when we hear people speak of the sick man's return to society, as if he had not been in his society whilst sick, especially if he has been in hospital. It is as if it is thought that human defects and illness do not belong to 'proper' life and that individuals who have by accident succumbed to the fate of being ill (or dying) are not actual, proper members of society unless they recover, unless they can be made healthy again.

Separation or segregation is effected by society in various ways; for example through physical barriers and through psychosocial barriers.

PHYSICAL BARRIERS

These barriers prevent interaction with the disabled and remain in most countries, although some countries have in recent years passed protective legislation to combat these discriminatory practices. Such legislation has included modification of architectural barriers in public buildings and, in some cases, even private houses.[7]

The main mobility problems encountered by the physically disabled are:

1. *mobility requirements in the home* — use of bathroom, toilets, and

kitchen which should be specifically adapted for wheelchair users;

2. *accessibility of public buildings* such as schools, theatres, museums, libraries, shopping centres and picture theatres;
3. *accessibility of recreational facilities* such as sports stadiums and vacation resorts;
4. *accessibility of means of transportation*, including planes, buses and parking places adjusted to the needs of disabled drivers.

Physical barriers definitely prevent integration of the disabled into society for a number of reasons, for example because:

(a) the disabled, by their non-presence in everyday life, are not seen by the larger population as having some special needs;
(b) the barriers prevent the disabled from social interaction, e.g. public toilets, as stated, are not suitable, and even friends' toilets are difficult or impossible to use.

The resulting forced social isolation frequently leads to feelings of depression and rejection, and has been reported as leading to psychological withdrawal in order to find some kind of emotional equilibrium.[8]

PSYCHOSOCIAL BARRIERS

In most societies, there persist a number of discriminatory practices which are basically based on prejudice. The reluctance to interact socially with the disabled has been reported by many researchers.[9] Such prejudice, which is called 'social' or 'affective', is probably the most deeply rooted one, and for this reason cannot be touched or modified by legislation.

Prejudice, being a multi-dimensional variable, results in discriminatory practices reflecting many degrees of intolerance for disabled people. These vary from a point at which people do not wish the disabled, especially the visibly disabled, to be present in public places, to unwillingness to rent them apartments, let them stay in motels, give them loans, insurance policies, drivers' licences, or admit them to normal schools and universities. Present changes in accessibility to places such as schools and universities do suggest that some shift in these discriminatory policies has occurred.

It has also been found that people may be willing to employ the disabled, yet be reluctant to interact socially with them beyond nominal acceptance.[10]

Discriminatory practice has not been equally distributed, for example:

some disabled people have been more stigmatised and isolated than others; visible disability consistently generates a greater amount of discrimination; facial disfigurements in particular, despite the fact that they do not necessarily cause functional impairment, set such people apart and bring about the need for discriminatory practices, particularly as such disfigurements tend to provoke fear and disgust.[11]

In the case of non-visible disability, it is the knowledge of its existence, certified by a doctor's official diagnosis, which triggers discrimination and intolerance. As long as the non-visible disability is not known about and the disabled person can pass for normal, he is accepted as such. However, in the case of MS, due to its deteriorating aspects, such a person cannot pass as 'normal' for long. This is in spite of the fact that people frequently develop a wide range of concealing techniques and tricks, which in themselves may often be painful, stressful or humiliating.

Once such a person's true identity (diagnosis) is uncovered, the seriousness of the discrimination depends on the nature and the assumed pervasiveness of the disability; whether or not it is contagious, considered hereditary and, as well, upon the degree and severity of the social stigma attached to it in the particular country in which that person is living.[12] Subsequent to recent reports of a viral cause of MS, some people have reported experiencing more rejection.

The severity of the disability and the degree to which its course can be predicted and controlled also seem to influence whether or not a disabled person will be helped, accepted or confined and isolated.[13] This has been evident in the case of MS, particularly in regard to the family response. An ongoing study is presently revealing that the family appears to develop a cut-off point where an attitude is developed in which the course of MS is no longer seen as even remotely controlled, even in the fluctuating MS sense, and can only be predicted in a downward mental slide. This attitude then results in rejection and eventual isolation or confinement of the affected MS family member.[14]

Stigmatisation

Stigmatisation, as a societal response to illness, affects the outcome of a person's adaptation to his illness. Monteiro[15] found, for example, that the objective nature of the disease episode, with regard to its severity and residual capacity, was in itself not sufficient to explain the cardiac patient's recovery behaviour. Neither the person who had had a heart attack nor his family saw the attack as something to be ashamed of or as something that 'spoils' the person's character. Such an absence of stigmatisation allowed the patient more latitude in his adaptation to his heart attack than other people had with stigmatised illness. However, people with MS in fact frequently feel ashamed of their disease and symptoms, and report family members or friends feeling similarly. Such feelings in MS frequently lead to defensive responses which in turn are seen by others as direct consequences of the illness rather than of the stigmatisation. This in turn further confuses the reactions of the non-disabled to people with disabilities.

Goffman[16] sums up some of the consequences of the stigmatising label:

> An individual who might have been received easily into ordinary social intercourse, possesses a trait that can obtrude itself upon attention and turn those of us whom he meets away from him, breaking the claim that his other attributes have upon us; he possesses a stigma, an undesired differentness from what we had anticipated . . . we believe the person with a stigma is not quite human; on this assumption, we exercise varieties of discrimination, through which we effectively, if often unthinkingly, reduce his life chances. We construct a stigma theory, an ideology to explain his inferiority . . . we tend to impute a wide range of imperfections on the basis of the original one . . . further, we may perceive his defensive response to his situation as a direct expression of his defect . . .

Effect on the Non-disabled

The non-disabled have been reported as feeling repulsion and disgust for the disabled, accompanied by guilt about these unacceptable feelings.[1] As a consequence of the conflict, avoidance of contact with the disabled is preferred. When contact is unavoidable, however, interaction tends to be strained and unreal. Relatives of MS-disabled persons have reported that they find it difficult to express anger or even feel anger towards the MS person, regardless of how irritating such a person's personality or offensive his behaviour can be.[5] Since the non-disabled tend to feel it necessary to watch their every gesture and words closely in order not to make a negative slip or show their aversion, and since norms regulating disabled and non-disabled interaction are quite ambiguous for both parties, such interactions are reported as uncomfortable, rigid and strained.[11]

The presence of a disabled person alone limits normal interaction in a whole host of ways and hence disables the non-disabled as well. Studies report that disability seriously affects the families of the disabled, both in restricting the range and flexibility of their activities due to the demands for help made by the presence of the disabled and by their acquisition of what Goffman has called 'courtesy stigma'. As has been seen in previous chapters in this book, by virtue of their close assocation with the disabled, their families may also become stigmatised. It is therefore not at all surprising that marked stress on marital relations is reported in regard to MS. A Brisbane study reports that if the wife had MS, her marriage appeared to fare better than if the husband had MS.[8] It was surmised that this was probably so, because the disabled status is more compatible with the traditional more passive role of ths woman who does not have to support the family. Since that report, however, it has also become clear, after therapy with the spouses of such women, that the dependent status of the disabled woman may inspire some insecure men who can comfortably play the protective role of the adequate and strong male.

DISABILITY AND MINORITY GROUP STATUS

A number of studies report that the disabled are essentially a minority group adapting to the larger society. However, this view has attracted some controversy. The disabled group does share with other minority groups some characteristics in societal reactions.

1. Interaction is encouraged with fellow-disabled only.
2. The majority of the non-disabled avoid contact with the disabled because they consider them to be inferior in many areas,[17] and use segregation as a means of keeping a considerable social and even territorial distance.
3. The segregation imposed by the majority of the non-disabled is rationalised by them as beneficial, as it is thought that with segregation the disabled have a better chance to find happiness and acceptance among their own kind than in the larger society. The disabled person here is encouraged to accept his disability (i.e. accept the fact that he is different from the 'normal' majority). Such an individual is seen as adjusted if he performs his social and vocational roles to the best of his ability, but restricts expression of his dissatisfaction of his emotional, social and psychological needs to his own disabled group.
4. There is a marked tendency to evaluate the disabled on the basis of their categorical membership more than on their individual characteristics. In other words, the disability trait overshadows and qualifies all other traits.

Such evaluation has also been noted with regard to MS, where people reported that once their diagnosis was known, people, instead of attempting a realistic assessment of their chronic condition, considered them to be in the same category as the worst MS condition, even though the person with MS still felt capable. On the other hand, others reported having been treated as though they possessed exceptional capacities and abilities, although those MS persons basically felt, and in fact were, fairly average at these capacities and abilities. For example, to be a doctor or a solicitor with MS and still perform one's duties resulted in a social reaction of awe and an over-evaluation of such a person's capacity in all other areas as well as the professional one. It appears that if a person is disabled, his disability covers all activities and potentialities in the eyes of a large number of non-disabled. Rarely, in fact, did people with MS report that they were evaluated objectively on the basis of their independent knowledge, abilities, skills, strengths and weaknesses. This is in keeping with reported reactions to other disabilities. Simons[14] reports that the non-disabled assess the disabled on the basis of the overall stereotype attached to all disabled as well as on the basis of the particular stereotype attached to their specific type of disability. Since these stereotypes are usually negative, the disabled are discriminated against by the non-disabled, particularly as the assessment stops at the recognition of the presence of the disability.

Although these reactions to disability are similar to those expressed to minority groups, there are differences as well. For example, some minority groups, such as southern Europeans, have at times been assigned undesirable characteristics that are seen by society as a result of a voluntary character (such as laziness, manipulativeness, unreliability, untrustworthiness, etc.). Such an attitude results in, or justifies, discriminatory reactions on behalf of the larger society.

In the case of disability, in particular with MS, where medical treatment has failed to eliminate the symptoms, the degree of responsibility that can be assigned to the MS-disabled for their present state is diminished or not able to be applied. A number of other factors have also been stated which clearly set disability apart from a minority group status. These have included the fact that ethnic groups, for example, have at least a primary group to which they can return for support. In contrast, the disabled have characteristics which, unlike a minority group, set them apart from their primary group and such characteristics not infrequently tend to result in losing the support of their primary group.

The common consequences of MS as a stigmatising illness can be summed up, then, in terms of how they relate to activity and to attitudes. In the area of activity, the physiological or functional incapacity leads to some restriction and restructuring of activity. However, there will also be a contraction in areas of social activity which is not directly attributable to the severity of the impairment but rather to the social construction of stigma. This curtailment results from the reluctance of others to interact with the individual and also from the individual withdrawing from the situation in which he might be rebuffed.[8] In extreme cases, stigmatising illness such as MS may result in the almost complete social isolation of the individual. The attitudes which result are more variable in strength and impact. For example, there are the attitudes towards oneself as somehow 'spoiled' and inferior. These are often coupled with feelings of uncertainty and inadequacy.

Looking further at society's reaction to disability, particularly the issue of segregation versus integration, it is clear that such an issue presents a complicated dilemma. Whilst segregation sounds inhuman, integration on present terms does not always appear desirable. For an MS-disabled person to become integrated in a so-called normal society, he will have to compete on an equal footing with the non-disabled. Not only will the MS-disabled have to adapt to a world made for the non-disabled, but he will have to do it on the non-disabled terms. It will clearly be more acceptable and easier if the non-disabled adapt and adopt at least some of the values and norms of the disabled. Each group, in other words, will have to accommodate the other partially to a point of more or less equal, mutual exchange.

It became clear that through the social acceptance and approval of other MS-disabled and through the identification with such a well-functioning and otherwise normal person, people with MS reported eventual acceptance of their disability and continued their lives with all the capacities that remained. However, it was also noted that the *crucial* social interaction was normally with the non-disabled. Therefore, integration appears to be an eventual '*must*' for the MS-disabled person.

The establishment of a normal interaction with the non-disabled is also of crucial importance to disablement other than MS. Such normal interaction reassures the involved disabled that he can be socially accepted despite his disability. Some researchers mention that extensive contact with disabled individuals diminishes the non-disabled degree of prejudice and results in less discrimination and in turn eases interpersonal relationships. However, not all contacts produce this effect and studies have shown that the results of the contacts depend upon their frequency, duration and variety.[18]

This chapter has attempted to show that people with MS, disabled under their multiple physical and social handicaps, encounter serious difficulties in adjusting to their disability. Their poor interpersonal relationships as a result of stigmatisation and other societal values are an additional and marked factor that impedes acceptance of the disability and real integration into society. It was also seen that society's reaction to disability affected the non-disabled in that it produced guilt feelings, family break-up, strained interpersonal relations and in many other ways disabled the non-disabled. It appears, therefore, to be to the benefit of the able and the disabled to reduce markedly, or eliminate, the negative reactions of society towards disablement. Past experience has shown that it is no use merely preparing the disabled to be integrated: the community's prejudices must be overcome and society at large persuaded to accept the disabled.[18] To overcome society's negative reaction to disability, it would appear that changing attitudes would be the best approach to this problem. Suggestions have been made to start attitude formation in schools at all levels and in integrated schools with the teachers as well as the students in order to prevent the formation of prejudices, at an early age. In fact, no means of publicity and education of the public in order to change attitudes should be neglected and the media, meetings of the public and of associations of parents and families of the disabled should be used. Also, it appears that thus far, special facilities in institutions have inhibited integration and, by shielding the public and the disabled from each other, have done nothing to change attitudes. Such facilities should therefore be thoroughly reviewed. Knowledge of the fact that these types of institutions inhibit integration should be incorporated into future planning of facilities for the disabled. It is as much on the part of some professionals as on the part of the general public and even some families involved to institute the changing in attitudes. Persons with disabilities in general themselves may provide the best answer to this problem, demonstrating that they are capable of making meaningful choices and participating in the social and economic life of their community to the extent of their abilities and the training and opportunities provided. In this regard, a self-advocacy movement is seen as crucial. In other words, a change should be made from voluntary organisations *for* disabled persons to organisations *of* disabled persons.

REFERENCES

1. Safilios-Rothschild C. (1970). *The Sociology and Social Psychology of Disability and Rehabilitation*, New York: Random Press.
2. Zahn M.A. (1973). Incapacity, impotence and invisible impairment: their effects upon interpersonal relations. *Journal of Health and Social Behaviour*; **14**:115.

3. Bersheid E., Walster E., Bohanstedt G. (1973). The happy American: a survey report. *Psychology Today*; **8**:119.
4. Murphy E., Johnson W.G. (1973). *The Effects of Disability on the Family*. Paper presented at the American Sociological Association Meetings, New York, September 1973.
5. Simons A.F. (1979). *Multiple Sclerosis: Not Just a Medical Condition*. Paper held by the Multiple Sclerosis Society of Queensland.
6. Fitzgerald R., ed. (1979), *The Sources of Hope*. Sydney: Pergamon Press.
7. Fact Sheets on Sweden (1980). *Support for the Handicapped in Sweden*.
8. Simons A.F. (1980). *Multiple Sclerosis: an Initial Study to Identify the Perceptions of Patients to Health Care Personnel and the Quality of their Life*. Unpublished Masters Thesis, held at the University of Queensland.
9. Tuckett D., ed. (1976). *Medical Sociology*. London: Tavistock.
10. Rosenbaum C., Katz S. (1980). Attitudes toward the physically disabled: beliefs and their evaluation. *International Journal of Rehabilitation*; **3**(1):15.
11. Comer R.J., Paliavin J.A. (1972). The effects of physical deviants upon face-to-face interaction: the other side. *Journal of Personal and Social Psychology*; **23**(1):33.
12. Gellmann W. (1973). Roots of prejudice against the handicapped. In *Readings in Rehabilitation Counselling* (Patterson C.H., ed.). Illinois: Stipes.
13. Fabrega H., Manning B.K. (1972). Disease, illness and deviant careers. In *Theoretical Perspectives on Deviants* (Douglas J.D., ed.) pp. 93–116. New York: Basic Books.
14. Simons A.F. (1981). *Changing Attitudes toward Disability*. IYDP Sporting Wheelies Seminar — Sport and Recreation for the Disabled. Brisbane, April 1981.
15. Monteiro L.A. (1973). After heart attack: behavioural expectations for the cardiac. *Social Science and Medicine*; **7**:555.
16. Goffman E. (1963). *Stigma: Notes on the Management of Spoiled Identity*. Englewood Cliffs, New Jersey: Prentice-Hall.
17. Bury M.R. (1979). Disablement in society: toward an integrated perspective. *International Journal of Rehabilitation*; **2**(1):33.
18. United Nations (1980). *Development of National Programmes for Integration of Disabled Persons into Community Life*. United Nations.

Recreation and Multiple Sclerosis

Ian Patterson is Lecturer in Community Recreation at the North Brisbane College of Advanced Education, Queensland. In this chapter he explains the importance of access to recreational pursuits to people with MS, and how involvement in such activities as sport, dance etc. can assist in meeting the social, psychological and physical needs of people disabled with MS.

He discusses the reasons why people with large amounts of leisure time due to disability are unable or unwilling to participate in available recreational activities and suggests ways in which recreational programmes can be planned to overcome the difficulties experienced.

Multiple sclerosis has been defined as a chronic debilitating disease of the central nervous system characterised by progressive exacerbations and remissions.[1] Although this disease exhibits a wide variety of neurological symptoms, its effects are generally physically disabling* for the sufferer. Its symptoms are usually characterised by various degrees of weakness, fatigue, inco-ordination, visual disturbance and difficulties in breathing, speech or swallowing.[2]

Therefore, the recreation worker must carefully consider the need to adapt and modify activities to suit the different physical conditions caused by MS. As well as the physical changes that occur, personality changes have also frequently occurred; so closely related as to make the changes inseparable. Therefore the objectives of any recreation programme should be to help satisfy the social and psychological needs as well as the physical needs of the person with MS.

* World Health Organization (in the United Nations, 1977) defined disabled persons as 'those persons whose physical and/or mental well being is temporarily or permanently impaired, whether congenitally or through age, illness or accident, resulting in an impediment to their self-dependence, schooling or employment.'

THE LEISURE NEEDS OF THE PHYSICALLY DISABLED

Authors such as Pomeroy[3] and Kraus[4] have been in agreement that the leisure needs of many physically disabled persons have been neglected in the past. It has only been in the last 15 years that people working in the field have become aware of the values of leisure experiences for the physically disabled: to improve socialisation and to increase social contacts; to develop self-confidence and individuality; and to provide opportunities for learning and personal experience. (For a much more comprehensive list of the goals of any recreation programme for the disabled, see Kraus.[5])

To define leisure and recreation is not simple. Many different versions of such definitions have been offered over time, and while many of these contain elements of similarity, many also are mutually exclusive. Leisure can be defined as:

> A state of mind which ordinarily is characterised by unobligated time and willing optimism. It can involve intensive activity or no activity. The key ingredient is an attitude which fosters a peaceful, productive coexistence with the elements in one's environment.

However, recreation has been defined slightly differently:

> Recreation is an attitude which is necessarily connected with productive self-satisfying and beneficial activity. It can occur in a number of areas: sport, art/craft, employment, community service, communion with nature and others. The key ingredient is a healthy outlook flowing from constructive activity which sustains, revitalizes and recreates the individual.[6]

Both leisure and recreation have been noted to have common elements:

1. free (unobligated) time;
2. activity which is carried out in unobligated time;
3. a state of mind; an attitude;
4. a cleaning or re-building of the mind and body, regardless of time and place.

Therefore leisure and recreation can be seen in concise terms as productive activity which sustains the individual, which is beneficial to all, and which fosters a spirit which enables the individual better to value and contribute to his environment and his society.

A disabled person is entitled to have the same human rights as everyone else, therefore he has the right to participate in and be introduced to all types of recreation activities during his leisure time.

Recreation experiences should be seen as a normal part of the physically disabled's daily lives and should not be seen as something separate, or as therapy which is done for specific purposes. The 1970 report of an enquiry made by the British Disabled Living Foundation into Sport and Physical Recreation for the Disabled stated:

> In common with all other members of the community, those who are disabled have every right to decide for themselves how to spend their time. But justice demands that the disabled no less than the able bodied should have adequate opportunities to take part in sporting activities if they wish to do so.

Pomeroy[3] and Calder[7] stress the need for constructive and creative recreation programmes, because of the large amounts of leisure time that many disabled persons have at their disposal.

Calder states 'disabled persons are often those who are normally faced with extensive periods of leisure but with limited opportunity to engage in appropriate recreation activities during their leisure.'

Calder has noticed that in Australia many disabled persons are still deprived of the right to develop to the fullest extent of their potential as they have fewer opportunities to learn leisure pursuits: '. . . that will add the dimension to life that such opportunities can afford'.[7]

In a small survey of MS sufferers carried out by the author[8] in Brisbane, Queensland, it was found that although 44.7% of persons interviewed who were suffering from MS had more than 40 hours of

Table 1 The amount of leisure time available to multiple sclerosis patients

Hours	Amount of leisure time per week		Amount of time spent in leisure pursuits	
	Number	Percentage	Number	Percentage
None			5	13.2
1–10	1	2.6	11	29.0
11–20	2	5.3	7	18.4
21–30	2	5.3	5	13.2
31–40	7	18.4	3	7.8
41+	17	44.7	4	10.6
No information	9	23.7	3	7.8
Total	38	100.0	38	100.0

leisure time, only a small amount of this time was actually spent in leisure pursuits (the largest group of MS sufferers— 29% — only spent between 1 and 10 hours in leisure pursuits; Table 1).

This supported the hypothesis that although the MS sufferer has a large amount of leisure time, very little of it is spent in actual leisure pursuits.

RECREATION AND SELF-CONCEPT

Matson and Brooks[9] were interested in finding out if the onset of MS would produce a negative effect on the individual's self-concept. They noted that the physical changes occurring with the onset of the disease were inextricably linked with personality changes.

Self-concept was defined as: 'The image one holds in one's minds eye of oneself—the awareness of one's various characteristics and one's evaluation of those characteristics.'[9] That is, self-concept is a person's perceptions of him or herself, which according to Goffman[10] undergoes continual changes as it is influenced by new circumstances. The lowering of self-concept by the MS sufferer involves a body image change which includes some acceptance of oneself as a disabled person and hence less of a 'real' person.

This attitude toward disabled persons can generally be attributed to society at large, and has been found to be inculcated from an early age.[11]

Matson and Brooks[9] found this to be the case in their exploratory study. As the disease brings on greater impairment and activity restrictions, the physical factor score of the self-concept decreases.

An increasing interest in leisure and recreation activities may be one means of helping ths MS sufferer to cope with his or her disease, and to assist in the rebuilding of the self-concept.

Nelson, a MS sufferer, in his book *Wheelchair Vagabond*,[12] found that travel opened up a new world to him:

> I spent years wallowing in the ugliness of self-pity, despair, sluggish awareness. Travel is what brought me out of my personal black pit. Vagabonding lifted me from the mud to the blue sky. I felt as Lazarus must have. I was reborn.

Therefore recreation and leisure services should ideally *help to develop, test and maintain the disabled person's own identity; to develop self-confidence and help to give a real sense of individuality, and these are important objectives for any leisure service*.

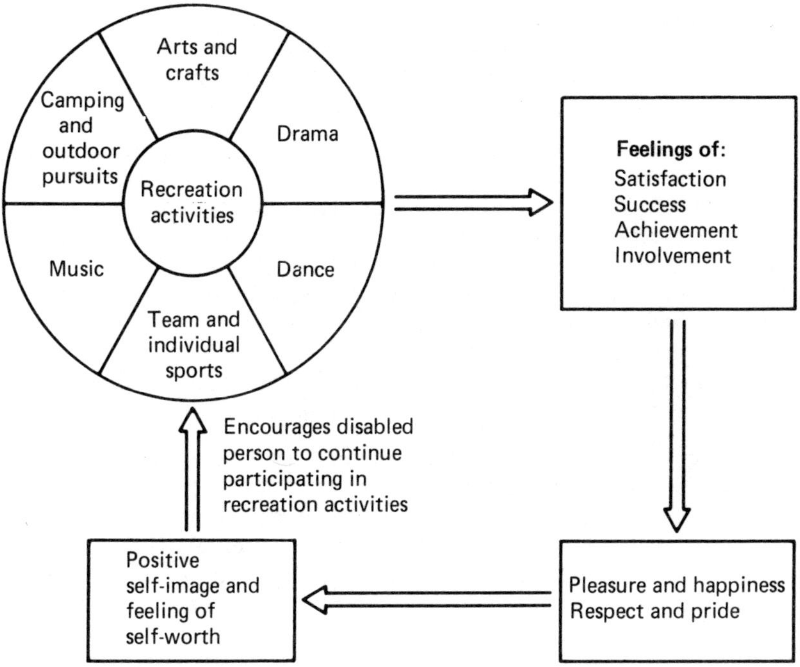

Fig. 1 Opportunities provided by recreation programmes.

Recreation has been defined by Gray[13] as:

> . . . an emotional condition within an individual human being that flows from a feeling of well being and satisfaction. It is characterised by feelings of mastery, achievement, exhilaration, acceptance, success, personal worth and pleasure. *It reinforces a positive self image*. Recreation is a response to aesthetic experience, achievement of personal goals or positive feedback from others.

Recreation programmes therefore need to provide opportunities for the physically disabled person to develop and maintain his or her own self-identity. Through the learning of new skills, the disabled person gains satisfaction and happiness which help to build up self-confidence and give a positive feeling of self-worth (Fig. 1).

Recreation is one aspect of life which perhaps provides us with the easiest obtainable opportunities for realising achievement, relaxation, respect, pride and self-worth.

Bob Douglas, an MS sufferer, explains how his major leisure pursuit, horse riding, played a major part in his rehabilitation:

> Horseback riding was always something I really liked. Before I had my remission I was in a wheelchair. But I found I could do one thing, no matter how bad I felt. I could still ride. When I was really down, feeling I couldn't handle things — something about being able to control a thousand pound animal renewed my strength. It gave me confidence that I could be a success at other things I needed to do.[14]

Physically disabled persons face enormous frustrations in living within a non-disabled world. The major problems are boredom, isolation and embarrassment, which all tend to discriminate against disabled persons. Recreation activities help to provide stimulation with the learning of new skills and thus may reduce boredom and isolation by supplying opportunities for becoming acquainted with new and interesting people.

RECREATION AND SOCIAL INTERACTION

Crandell[15] stated that social interaction is an important motivator for participation in leisure activities, and as a source of satisfaction derived from them. In fact, Crandell concluded that social interaction may be as important in the enjoyment of many leisure activities as the facilities or activities themselves:

> People . . . want the satisfaction which comes not so much from an

> activity itself as from the opportunity for close group association. The activities in which they engage are thus incidental to their need for group association.[16]

Calder[17] noted that disabled teenagers interviewed during the Youth Action Project stated that their greatest need was for the opportunity to meet and make friends and to be involved in activities away from their particular institution.

Therefore recreation and leisure services should *help improve socialisation and increase interaction with other persons*.

Interaction is essential if personality growth is to occur. Without interaction with other people, the disabled individual cannot develop his or her ideas, thoughts and attitudes and has little chance of self-understanding. Recreation programmes allow the physically disabled person to learn the skills of interaction and the opportunities to practise these skills. Hercox *et al*.[18] found, in their dance group of MS patients at the Vanderbilt Clinic, that many of the women came dressed for a social occasion. During sessions they frequently exchanged information and helpful suggestions. Conversations ranged from how to cope with depressions to where to buy wigs and clothes, since they must shop by mail order. After class they wheeled to the coffee shop together.

Carpenter[19] summed his feelings up by stating:

> The main handicap that a disabled person has is not his physical disability but rather his lack of social development. For this reason recreation for the physically disabled . . . should not perpetuate the sheltered environment concept, but try to break the over-protective cycle by gearing recreational programmes to promoting integration between the two groups in our society: the 'normal' and 'disabled'.

Therefore recreation and leisure services should ideally *help to integrate the disabled person into the mainstream of community life*.

Many disabled persons who live in institutional settings have limited opportunities for individual achievement, and are generally unaware of the recreational opportunities available in the community. Carpenter[19] concluded that integration is more difficult for physically disabled adults, because they become accustomed to routine and set patterns of living, and find it almost impossible to change their life-styles. Martens and Bacon[20] found this to be the case, in a small study of MS patients at Granston Lodge in Brisbane, Queensland. They found that many preferred to engage in recreational activities with other MS patients within the centre itself, because they were relieved of any concern or embarrassment about their disability. The main reasons given for not wanting to be involved in outside community visits and activities were:

1. fatigue — many tired easily and did not like going on long trips;
2. their disabilities generally ruled out involvement in physical activities;
3. embarrassment in doing fine craft work due to tremor or spasticity;
4. lack of transport and accessibility to facilities in general;
5. many found it very time consuming to arrange transport and enquire about accessibility in organising trips outside the centre.

Therefore Martens and Bacon concluded that many people with MS slip into voluntary withdrawal from integrated community activities. In their study this was due mainly to the sudden loss of freedom and continual dependence upon others, as well as the embarrassment caused by their disability and the negative attitude of outsiders. They enjoyed the relationships established at the Multiple Sclerosis Society, but were not prepared to be involved with people outside in the community. This was because of the hassles involved in organising trips and visits and the embarrassment caused by their disabilities. Therefore it seems that the constant difficulties, frustrations and failures coupled with social rejection are highly significant factors contributing to apathy or poor self-esteem with physically disabled persons.

Recreation and leisure services should be organised with an *awareness that physically disabled people are faced with a variety of environmental barriers which may prevent them from meeting their recreational needs*.

Architectural barriers present major access problems for physically disabled persons — stairs, door widths, and toilet facilities often are not considered when providing community recreation programmes for disabled persons. In America, national parks are now being made accessible for wheelchairs and to those who are blind. Features include:[21]

1. gently sloping wide, paved trails and paths and paved walkways to toilets;
2. picnic tables and spaces for wheelchairs;
3. low drinking fountains and taps;
4. fishing piers protected with guard rails; and
5. rest rooms without entrance steps, or with ramps and handrails; enough space beside to manoeuvre wheelchairs, cubicles with wide doors; hand rails and benches; and special clothes-hanging facilities.

The availability of transportation is also a most crucial factor in determining whether or not disabled persons get out into the community. Provision is being made to assist physically disabled persons to travel by air in comfort and many drive their own cars. The majority, however, are dependent upon the good will of other people or parents and friends for transportation to recreation programmes.

Financial barriers are another important factor in preventing physically disabled persons being involved in recreation programmes. The income from disabled persons' pensions provides only a basic subsistence living; whereas expenses may be quite high for such things as medical supplies, special appliances, wheelchairs etc. This generally leaves very little over for spending on recreation outings and activities.

Recreation and leisure services should *provide an enjoyable physical outlet for the physically disabled, through a properly supervised exercise programme which aims to improve physical ability by achieving gains in such areas as strength, co-ordination and balance*.

Hardy and Cull[22] found that a physical exercise programme is a vital factor in helping MS sufferers adjust to their disability. Through the use of a bilateral system of pulleys, patients are taught to perform exercises for their upper and lower extremities. They conclude by stating:

> Our experience over the past eighteen years has found that multiple sclerosis patients on a functional exercise programme that meets individual needs, progress far better than the patients who remain confined to a wheelchair or bed. These patients on a total rehabilitation programme maintain a high level of well-being, experience fewer exacerbations and are able to maintain their functional level.[22]

It is important that exercise programmes are appropriately tailored to the individual's medical status, needs and problems. Fatigue must be carefully avoided as MS lessens motor power for a longer period of time and to a greater degree than is usually seen in other illnesses. Professor Russell[23] developed and claimed success for a rest and exercise programme (REP). He based it on the theory that the lesions of MS are caused or influenced by areas of circulatory insufficiency in the white matter of the central nervous system. He found that exercises must be adapted to the particular type of disability. If the MS sufferer is not disabled, running, skipping, cycling, sports and gardening or exercise on a rowing machine are added to the daily programme. However, Russell advised the need for short periods of 10 to 20 minutes rest, lying down at least two or three times during the day. The most vigorous part of the exercises is done with the upper limbs — this encourages a response in the blood circulation to the upper spinal cord and brainstem. The main types of exercises suggested are press-ups, weight lifting, and the use of springs.

Dance has also been used as a means of physical rehabilitation for MS sufferers. Hercox *et al.*[18] organised an MS group at Vanderbilt Clinic,

Columbia-Presbyterian Medical Center. There were five wheelchair-bound women in the group of seven. Dance sessions emphasised what one could do, rather than striving to correct what one could not do. To aid in function, movement dynamics such as swinging and counter-balance were taught, as well as substitute movements from the hip when the thigh could not do it. Emphasis was on the use of areas not severely affected neurologically, but weak from disuse, therefore seeking to maintain the range of motion and strength. *All participants reported an increase in function*.

THE ROLE OF THE RECREATION WORKER WITH THE PHYSICALLY DISABLED

The recreation worker needs to encourage the abilities of physically disabled people so that they will be involved in a wide programme of activities which encourage self-expression, social involvement and creative experiences. However, the recreation worker needs to be aware that involvement should be voluntary, and that not all physically disabled people are ready to participate in all activities. Therefore it is important that the recreation worker helps to eliminate any feelings of concern and threat; whereas if the disabled person experiences success, it will help to develop and generate confidence and self-respect.

The recreation worker should encourage the disabled person's right to take risks. To shield him from risk taking is unfair and unrealistic:

> The single most important point made by those interviewed was the difficulty the handicapped face in participating in various recreation programmes because of the fears and limited imaginations of the able bodied who work with them.[24]

Carpenter[19] also felt that over-protectiveness was one of the major factors in limiting the self-identity of many disabled persons. He makes the point that many parents shield their children from the cruel society which might laugh at or scorn them if they went out in public.

Therefore the recreation worker should provide opportunities to develop and practise skills to build up self-confidence so as to create a positive self-image (Fig. 2).

Meserow[25] outlined four major principles of recreation programming for the physically disabled person.

1. Programmes should consist of meaningful, personally gratifying experiences.

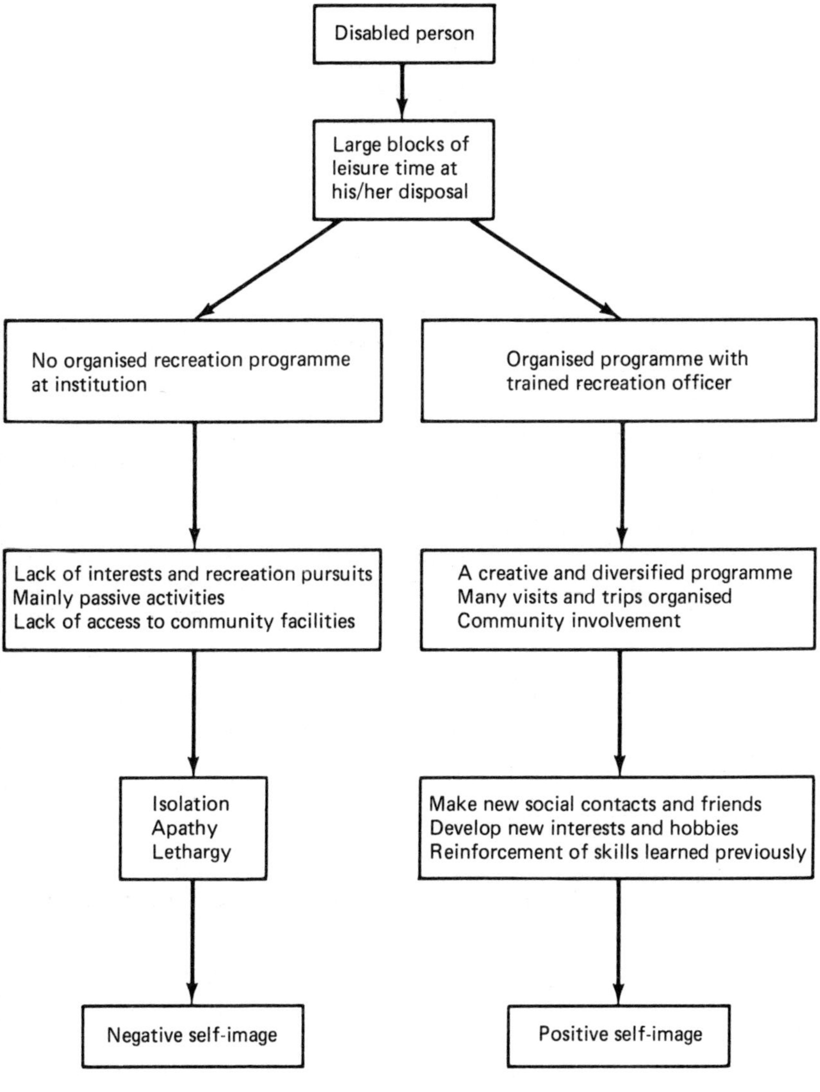

Fig. 2 Comparisons of factors leading to the development of a negative or a positive self-image.

2. Programmes should promote independence, confidence, self-esteem, pleasure and above all the element of choice.
3. Programmes should be aimed at integrating the disabled person into the general community as much as possible.
4. Programmes should accept the responsibility for risks and challenges, for without challenges man 'atrophies'.

The following are pointers when planning recreation activities for the MS sufferer.

1. Plan any travel or trip well in advance. Survey the architectural barriers that may exist.
2. Plan any trip to avoid unnecessary fatigue. Do not leave at unusual hours or travel too far without the opportunity for rest.
3. Activities need to be adjusted or realistically modified to suit individual needs.
4. Set a balance between rest and activity and acquire knowledge and understanding of changes if they occur.

Leisure experiences should be seen as a normal part of the disabled person's life, and are affected by all else that happens to the person. However, many disabled people are often faced with extensive periods of leisure which give rise to feelings of lethargy, frustration and uselessness; but opportunities to participate in outdoor leisure activities are often limited.

A creative and diversified recreation programme is vital to provide constructive activity to fill much of the disabled person's free time. As well as this there is a need to provide opportunity for growth to the fullest extent of the physically disabled person's capabilities: to meet and enjoy new friends, to develop new hobbies, to reinforce skills learned at school and to have the opportunity of experiencing new activities.

There is also a need for the disabled person to become aware of and use the community's resources. Being confined to an institution should not mean that the person is completely isolated from society. Pressure must be applied to management to provide adequate recreation programmes so as to allow the disabled person to develop to his or her fullest potential.

What are days for?
Days are where we live,
They come, they wake us
Time and time over.
They are to be happy in!
Where can we live but days?[26]

REFERENCES

1. Fouston M. (1967). *A Textbook of Neurology*, 4th edn. New York: Arlington House.
2. Braunel L., James C., Stovall J. (1979). *MS is a Family Affair*. Chicago: National Easter Seal Society for Crippled Children and Adults.
3. Pomeroy J. (1964). *Recreation for the Physically Handicapped*. Englewood Cliffs. New Jersey: Prentice Hall.
4. Kraus R. (1977). Therapeutic Recreation Service: past and present. In *Recreation Today: Program Planning and Leadership*, 2nd edn., pp. 1–32. California: Goodyear.
5. Kraus R. (1978). *Therapeutic Recreation Service: Principles and Practices*, 2nd edn. Philadelphia: W.B. Saunders.
6. RAIPR/ACHPER (1980). *Policy Document on Recreation*. Adelaide.
7. Calder J. (1974), *Recreation Accessibility for the Handicapped*. Paper presented at the National Seminar: Leisure— A New Perspective, Canberra, April 1974. Canberra: AGPS.
8. Patterson I. (1981). The leisure needs of the disabled. *Australian Journal of Health, Physical Education and Recreation*; **91**:33.
9. Matson R.R., Brooks N.A. (1977). Adjusting to multiple sclerosis: an exploratory study. *Journal of Social Science and Medicine*; **11**:245.
10. Goffman E. (1963). *Stigma*. Englewood Cliffs, New Jersey: Prentice Hall.
11. Simons A. (1978). *Multiple Sclerosis: Not Just a Medical Condition*. Paper held by the Multiple Sclerosis Society of Queensland.
12. Nelson J. (1975). *Wheelchair Vagabond. A Guide and Goad for the Handicapped Traveller*. Santa Monica, Calif: Project Press.
13. Gray D. (1972). Exploring inner space. *Parks and Recreation*; **7**:18.
14. Lattin D. (1975). Not just horsing around. *Performance*; **25**(9):9.
15. Crandell R. (1979). Social interaction, affect and leisure. *Journal of Leisure Research*; **11**(3):165.
16. Brightbill C. (1948). Group work in public recreation. In *A Decade of Group Work* (Hendry C.E., ed.) pp. 17–25. New York: Association Press.
17. Calder J. (1975). *Recreation — New Directions of the 70s*. Paper presented at the Australian Association of Occupational Therapists, Melbourne, August, 1975.
18. Hercox B., Levine E., Scott D. (1975). A report on the use of dance in physical rehabilitation. *Rehabilitation Literature*; **36**(1):5.
19. Carpenter R. (1976). Integration, self concept and recreation. *Leisuribility*; **3**(3):31.
20. Martens R., Bacon J. (1980). *Recreation for the Multiple Sclerosis Sufferer: Integration of Segregated*? Unpublished research paper for adaptive recreation course at North Brisbane College of Advanced Education, November 1980.
21. Stone E.H. (1971). There's a wheelchair in the woods. *Parks and Recreation*; **vi**(12):19.
22. Hardy R.E., Cull J.C. (1974). *Mental Retardation and Physical Ability*.

Illinois: Charles C Thomas.

23. Birrer C. (1979). *Multiple Sclerosis: a Personal View*. Illinois: Charles C Thomas.
24. The handicapped speak about their recreation needs (1974). *Trends*; p. 5.
25. Meserow P. (1975). *Recreation and People with an Orthopaedic Disability*. Paper presented at Seminar— Workshop for the Orthopaedically Handicapped at Tallebudgera National Fitness Camp, Queensland, September 1975.
26. Larkin Phillip (1965). Days. In *The Faber Book of Modern Verse* (Roberts M., ed.) p. 367. London: Faber & Faber.

A SIMONS

Perceptions of Health Care

Because of the variety of professions involved in the care of people with MS and the variable factors concerned in the disease itself, the evaluation of the 'success' of care varies depending on one's particular viewpoint.

In this chapter, a survey of patients at an MS centre in Australia is described, which attempted to assess how the respondents perceived the health care they received. The author describes the therapies available at the centre and the expectations and reactions to them of the respondents in the study. He finishes the chapter with some recommendations on how the specialist care of people with MS could be improved in the light of the study described.

Multiple sclerosis is now gaining attention not only from health care professionals but also from the general public in several countries. Reasons for this attention include changes in illness and disease distribution,[1] and the increased public visibility of disabled people, including those suffering from MS. Stressing both the cure and care needs of people with MS, television advertisements backed by people of world fame and MS Read-a-thon competitions at secondary schools have propelled MS into public view.

However, there appears to be a lack of consensus as to what constitutes 'good' or 'successful' care. This lack of consensus is not surprising, since care is a process involving doctors, nurses, occupational therapists, physiotherapists, psychotherapists, social workers, speech therapists, families, friends, government and the MS people themselves. In this regard, Katz[2] reported physiotherapists, for example, as viewing success in terms of increased levels of physical function, whereas occupational therapists perceived success in terms of improvements in skill levels necessary for physical independence and task performance. On the other hand, families and friends were reported as perceiving success in terms of how much the person's disability disrupted his life.[3] Therefore, such differing viewpoints of successful care appear largely to depend on the perspective of the participant. Few researchers have examined consumer perceptions of success, although they, as consumers of health care, might well be the best judges.[4, 5, 6]

Health care, particularly in regard to MS, involves numerous professions as a result of differences in deterioration rate, site of disability, premorbid personality and many other factors. Each health profession's view is likely to be biased in that health profession's favour. Evaluation of success, therefore, ought to take into account all viewpoints, including those of the MS person, if a more balanced view is to be obtained.

An investigation of the views of people suffering from MS was therefore carried out at an Australian MS centre and was concerned with the attitudes of people with MS toward the professional services provided for them at this centre. This centre, architecturally designed to minimise mobility problems, has a wide range of professional staff ranging from part-time doctors, full- and part-time nursing staff, an occuptional therapist, physiotherapists, a consulting psychologist, a full-time social worker and a full-time speech therapist, and has 41 beds catering for both long- and short-term admissions.

An attempt was made to ascertain how people with MS, who present as consumers of the above services, perceived the providers of their health care; which professional help they valued most; and what improvements they could recommend to make such professional help more useful and beneficial for their specific needs. Also investigated were issues dealing with the general quality of their lives.

It is to be stressed here that the results obtained were based on a pilot sample of 60 people with MS only. Also, that results may not accurately portray respondents' perceptions of health professionals in general, as the survey explored people's perceptions of their personal health professionals at this centre only. It has been demonstrated in this regard, that people are more likely to hold positive views about personal physicians, for example, than about the medical profession in general.[7] The image of the profession, in other words, may be poor, even though the evaluation of the personal health professionals may be the case in point.

FROM FAMILY TO HEALTH SPECIALIST SUPPORT

In MS, the stress of present health delivery is clearly on care and support rather than cure, which is often stressed by other diseases. Two sources from which care and support could come and were sought by people with MS in this study were found to be the person's family and health professionals in general. Initially relying on the family and the family doctor, it was found by most that the disease process of MS created an increasing need for health care intervention. With progressive deterioration, the family alone was not successful in helping the person with MS cope with his changing circumstances. To stay physically independent for as long as possible as well as learning to cope with the totality of the disease, the person with MS had to rely on increasing help from the health specialists.

FAMILY AND MARRIAGE

The impact of MS clearly produced marked changes in the quality of life. The importance of families in making life worthwhile, for example, was reported by over half of the respondents. Few, however, included their spouses in the family concept. Divorce, separation and near separation were reported as common. Looking at disability in general, a lack of consensus in the literature on the effect of disability on family life was reported.[8] For example, some workers found divorce rates were no higher among families with disabled members than among other families.[9]

In a study on patients on haemodialysis, marital relations were reported as not having undergone any great deterioration.[10] In some cases, in fact, the illness was reported as having led to even closer relationships. By contrast, another report indicated that disability was associated with high divorce rates.[11]

The present study and that of Lilius *et al*.[12] indicate the impact of MS leading to both high divorce and separation rates. These high rates appear to be attributable to a number of factors, including unrealistic expectations held toward the MS-disabled spouse, particularly as far as energy levels are concerned, income loss, sexual disturbances, and the general uncertainty about the progression of the disease and the near-normal life-span associated with the disease. Disruptions in the established role sets were reported by many in this study. Resulting feelings of humiliation, tension and guilt appeared to be common. The reported role disruptions were felt by the person with MS to be one of the more serious strains of familial adjustment to MS, particularly as they made them feel inadequate. Unrealistic expectations of spouses toward the capabilities of the MS person were given as creating marital tensions and were felt to be difficult to handle, due to the reported fluctuations in energy levels and the reported lack of knowledge on MS by the non-affected spouse. Refusal by the non-affected spouse to become involved led to reported feelings of rejection and depression. The family, in particular the spouse, was reported by many persons with MS either to impede their process of learning to cope, either by doing too many things for them or denying problems, or by not wanting to talk about MS and its impact on their relationships.

Similar findings were reported in relation to disablements other than MS.[13] These types of findings do raise the question as to whether the family is the best source of help for the MS person. At present, the family's help is sought, but they appear to be unwilling, unable or not knowledgeable enough to give this help, according to a high percentage of respondents in this study. Most MS-disabled people, in fact, reported that the best source of help came from the health professionals.

WORK

Marital problems included the already reported rejecting behaviour on the part of the non-MS spouses and sexual problems leading to frustrations. It was found, however, that married women with MS, particularly with children, reported fewer marital problems than married males with MS. Safilios-Rothschild,[11] stating similar findings for disabilities other than MS, reported that men were usually not accepted by their wives unless they could still perform the breadwinner role. The loss of this role was reported by males in this study as producing feelings of insecurity in themselves and rejecting behaviour in their wives. Findings also indicated that where the woman's primary role was that of mother and housekeeper, fewer role disturbances were reported. The basic tasks involved in such a role could still be reasonably performed even when the person with MS was markedly disabled. By contrast, the tasks and requirements of the breadwinner role were found to be generally disturbed by physical and mental aspects of MS, leading to the breadwinner losing his role.

It was found that the marriages of older men were stable despite disability because their wives, freed from child rearing, were able and willing to take over the breadwinner role.[14] However, this does not appear to be applicable to MS. Most of the older married men with MS in this study had grown-up children and working wives, yet most reported 'shaky' marriages and the possibility of early divorce or separation.

Thus far, it appears that males, having lost the breadwinner role as a result of MS, reported most difficulties in themselves, their family and society in general. Losing their jobs appears to diminish their own self-worth and also that of their spouses, both expressing this in a variety of ways, including social withdrawal. Where the respondent was a housewife, particularly with children, she appeared to feel only somewhat diminished in her self-worth and did not report social withdrawal of self or her family. The husband of such a woman with MS also, rather than being diminished, may simply be seen by society as shouldering an extra burden. Problems associated with losing the breadwinner role appeared in fact to be a central component in the quality of life of people with MS.

SOCIAL WITHDRAWAL

Factors leading to social isolation of the person with MS or his family were those of excessive fatigue, the long time periods needed to get ready to go out, pretending to feel 'normal', having social interaction which was not accepted as such by the non-disabled, the inability to find usable toilets, transport problems, the felt embarrassment of having to rely on others to carry things upstairs and thus becoming the focus of attention, unsteady gait and sphincteric disturbances. These and others were all reported to lead to a 'preferred' social withdrawal on that person's part. Some reported having tried to escape the 'deviance' stigma by acting 'normal'. However, fatigue, disappointment and unchanged or even increased stigmatisation were experienced as a result of these attempts and had led them to give up their re-integrating efforts with the non-disabled. Feeling nearly continuously rejected by the non-disabled, they were becoming somewhat emotionally 'deviant' by withdrawing completely in order to find some kind of emotional equilibrium.

Many more changes in themselves, family and others were reported, and indicated MS as severely affecting the quality of their lives and that of their family and friends. Physical and psychosocial consequences of MS, some unique, others common to a variety of disabilities, led to eventual searching for increased help from some or all of the rehabilitation specialists.

SEXUAL

Where reported, respondents mentioned lack of sexual interest due to loss of orgasm either through fear of failing or just markedly reduced libido. Sexual problems are reported as commonly part of MS.[15, 16, 17] In the present study, some non-MS partners expressed a fear of 'getting MS' themselves as a result of intercourse. Such a fear resulted in rejecting the advances of the MS partner who interpreted this rejection as a personal one and reacted with hostility or withdrawal. Proper sexual counselling led to an improved sexual life within a few weeks for most.

Sexual changes for whatever reasons were reported by Lilius *et al.*[12] for 91% of males. In over half of their sample, interest in sexual intercourse was diminished or absent. Interpretation of their data indicated that the partner suffers more from disturbances in sexual life than does the person with MS. Such a finding is substantiated by current research in Brisbane, which states that the high frequency of divorce in MS found in a study carried out there may in some cases be attributable to spouses replacing impotent partners with sexually potent ones.

MALE/FEMALE DIFFERENCES IN SEEKING HELP

The number of females attending the centre on a daily basis in this study was found to be well above that of the average number of males attending on a daily basis. It was found in this regard that males were more resistant than females to entering a dependent role with health professionals.[18] The present study, as will be seen later, indicates that males did request earlier physiotherapy and psychotherapy.

These findings may still explain the differences in accepting care from other health professionals. It may be that physiotherapy and psychotherapy offer treatment allowing for more independent behaviour outside the treatment than other health professions provide, thereby reducing or eliminating the resistance to accepting assistance from both physiotheraphy and psychotherapy. The same authors also described the feminine gender role as being more congruent with the sick role than the masculine role.[18]

The study described in this chapter appears to substantiate the above findings further in that MS-disabled males reported their dependence as little tolerated by their wives, felt uneasy in themselves entering this role and also reported high guilt feelings, both psychologically and socially, as they also felt devalued in such role reversal. Females, by contrast, reported no such difficulties in relation to their increased dependency.

FINANCIAL

Income loss was experienced, particularly by those families in which the person with MS was the breadwinner. The incomes in these families were frequently reduced to pension level. Increased spending was reported by some and attributed to alterations (including widening of doorways and ramps) as well as purchase of equipment to facilitate the MS person's mobility. Financial pressures, changed life-styles, concomitant guilt feelings of the breadwinner and physical disabilities clearly placed considerable stress on families in which one partner had MS.

PERCEPTIONS OF HEALTH CARE PROFESSIONALS

The Doctor

Prior to seeing the doctor at the centre, a surprising number of people with MS had wishful expectations of this doctor, hoping to obtain a cure, or the next best thing — finding that the previous diagnosis of their conditon was incorrect! Although none regarded the medical intervention as a cure for their condition, they obtained some relief through drugs and some reduction in symptoms. However, the majority appeared to have other reasons for seeing the doctor, including just wanting company, reassurance on symptoms and how to obtain a housing commission home.

Similar findings were obtained in another study in which the doctor was not simply viewed as someone to remove the threat of illness or symptoms, but was also seen as someone who could solve other problems.[19]

Dependence on the doctor for reassurance was clear, as was a fear of being rejected by him if they 'bothered' him with 'silly' symptoms, thereby taking up his valuable time. The doctor was also seen as busy, which prompted some not to seek advice even where that advice could have alleviated anxiety. It has been reported in fact that when doctors gave the impression of being busy, patients tended to be less likely to seek advice.[20] Those people with MS who wanted reassurance requested regular contact *initiated* by the doctor. This type of contact appeared to be aimed at avoiding having to ask for help as well as providing a more natural setting to discuss possible 'silly' symptoms.

Nursing Care

Consumers of this service viewed this care as clearly more concerned with the everyday realm of activities than any other profession at the centre and were aware of their near-continuous involvement with it. Not surprisingly, therefore, the most recommended improvements were related to the concept of dependence and institutionalisation. Making them feel less aware of their dependence on the nursing staff and hence of their 'sick' status as well as reducing signs of institutionalisation by accepting individuality, were judged to be more important. 'Doing things my way' rather than the institutionalised way was a frequent comment. To be there when needed without being over-protective, as suggested by some, might well describe the wanted ideal type of nurse.

Occupational Therapy

'Something to do' and 'a social outlet' were the major reported differences derived from occupational therapy. 'Something to do' related to physical activities such as craft work or pottery, while the social outlet appeared to be related to psychosocial benefits obtained through sharing meals and coffee breaks in the occupational therapy centre. Although craft work gave certain people a sense of achievement and satisfaction, none commented on person-to-person relationships within the framework of occupational therapy activities which helped them gain an understanding of, or modify if necessary, some particular patterns of behaviour. Although re-education in such pursuits as housework, cooking, shopping and beauty care is provided by that occupational therapy department, it was commented on by only one female who appreciated the cooking practice. Those who found occupational therapy helpful reported that specific activities appeared to have stopped their 'shakes'. In this regard, re-education of affected muscle groups was reported by Fidler and Fidler[21] as being one of the major functions of occupational therapy, with respect to physical disability. This function was fulfilled in the eyes of those who found this treatment helpful.

Females more than males and, not surprisingly, those in hospital more than those who attended the centre daily, commented on the social aspects of occupational therapy. Males in general though reported dissatisfaction. Such male dissatisfaction has also been reported by other researchers in a variety of occupational therapy settings. For example, it was reported that occupational care was regarded by males as mainly catering for females.[22] Although not reported by males in this study as such, it appeared to underly some of their comments. One male in particular, whose work identity had been that of a 'good provider' and whose work had brought in steady wages, felt occupational therapy to be 'women's fiddling and a waste of time'. Problems associated with work identity and the work concept were highlighted in occupational therapy. For example, one male requested more structured activities which included the concept of structured time. This aspect of the work concept was sadly missed by him.

On balance, it appears doubtful that occupational therapy convinced people with MS in this study that it is effective in helping them cope with their disease. Those who did obtain benefits though, did so through a clear understanding of benefits which could be derived from certain activities. In fact, most recommended that clear explanations be given to them as to why they should do certain tasks.

Physiotherapy

Physiotherapy was clearly seen as the most beneficial health intervention. Most started physiotherapy with high expectations of improving their physical abilities and seeing these expectations fulfilled or reduced to still acceptable physical benefits.

For some people with MS though, feelings toward physiotherapy care appeared to be ambiguous. They felt that with earlier physiotherapy they could have retained their independence a lot longer or, as one put it, 'delay the inevitable', whereas others stated that strenuous exercise had led to a deterioration in their MS condition. In this regard, physiotherapy and energy levels appeared to cause the most frequent clashes. For example, some reported days of needed recuperation after one day of physiotherapy. In fact, some requested termination of physiotherapy altogether. One person with MS commented 'Close the department altogether, I don't think physiotherapy helps MS one bit. It puts us in a wheelchair faster I think'.

Some older hospitalised people with MS complained that physiotherapists tended to view them as lost causes because of their age and condition, a reaction not uncommon in aged patients and, at times, firmly based in reality.[11] Some who attended on a daily basis suspected those who were hospitalised received better care, and some hospitalised people with MS suspected that those attending on a daily basis received the extra attention. These feelings of rejection, hostility and jealousy are not surprising when one considers the generally high value placed on physiotherapy. Even those who felt that physiotherapy was actually producing some deterioration of their condition would not report this to the therapist, hoping that continued therapy could still result in improvement.

Mostly, males with MS regretted the lack of earlier physiotherapy, feeling that it would have helped them stay independent longer. There was a trend obtained which indicated males entered physiotherapy earlier than did females. Such a trend appeared to confirm the earlier finding that dependent behaviour in males is less tolerated by family and friends, thereby leaving them little choice but to accept early health care and support from rehabilitation personnel, particularly physiotherapy. By contrast, females, because of their gender role, had their increased dependence tolerated by family and friends longer, before they too had to seek professional care in the form of physiotherapy.

Psychotherapy

It has been observed that: 'All occupations in the human relations field have only tenuous claims to exclusive competence'. This results not only from their 'newness', uncertain standards and the embryonic state of social and psychological sciences on which they draw, but also from the fact that the types of problems dealt with are part of everyday living. The lay public cannot recognise the need for special competence in an area 'where everyone is expert'. At this centre, however, people with MS clearly separated the psychologist from other professionals, particularly in terms of solving emotional problems within themselves and their families.

Psychotherapy was reported as beneficial by all and was reported by many as something they would have liked to have had earlier in their illness. Some reported psychotherapy as the most helpful intervention in the course of their illness. The benefits of psychotherapy commented on included: better communication at home; improved sexual lives; less guilt feelings about the impact of the disease; and, in some cases, the therapy was considered to lead to a less stressful divorce.

The positive response to psychotherapy at the centre is attributed to the type of therapy offered, which is thought to be acceptable to the MS condition and the social background of the average MS-disabled person at the centre. For example, it was found that working-class psychotherapy users dropped out of treatment more readily than middle-class ones due to working-class attitudes to life, lack of future-oriented perspective and an emphasis on tangible goals.[23] Although most people with MS attending this centre did not come from working-class families, it was found that their attitudes to the disease, including the deteriorating aspects of it, made the future-oriented perspective also less palatable to them. Such future-oriented perspective would often lead to the preparatory anxiety and depression, as discussed in Chapter 1.

A psychotherapy programme focusing on day-to-day problems with tangible goals was therefore offered to them. The high satisfaction rate and the *understood goals* of the psychotherapy produced a not unexpected near lack of views as to suggested improvements, with more help wanted in family matters being the only suggestion given.

Social Work

The most surprising aspect of social work was the near-total lack of expectation of the possible benefits of social work. The initial expectation, where expressed, was a desire to obtain information on social activities available to people with MS in the community. This expectation was reported as not fulfilled. Again, a number expressed the attitude of not wishing to ask for this information, seeing such behaviour as dependent and also as inviting possible rejection by the social worker. Main benefits, where derived from social work contact, were the reported guidance in such matters as social services, pensions and other available services from 'the system'. A few females reported the female social worker helpful in solving personal 'girl' problems. Recommending that the social worker should listen and explain, rather than 'tell us what to do', as some stated, might merely reflect social class differences between them and the social worker. In this regard, communication difficulties have been reported between social worker and 'client', both having been described as having very little idea 'what the other was on about'.[24] What was seen as a request by the 'client' was seen as a command by the social worker, and vice versa. Although the centre's social worker carried out case work with their families, none reported on this function. Further research into this aspect of the social work role in relation to MS, particularly considering the high divorce and separation rates obtained in this study, is indicated.

Speech Therapy

Speech therapy was reported by most as a very 'straightforward' rehabilitation care offered at the centre. Most expected their speech to improve and reported this expectation fulfilled.

Those who would have liked earlier speech therapy felt that improved speech would have saved social embarrassments, and complained that general practitioners had never referred them to a speech therapist, even though they had obviously needed such assistance. Such comments came mainly from females. The lack of males requesting earlier intervention may be due to the small sample taken, or may indicate that females feel more stigmatised by speech problems.

Satisfaction with speech therapy was high. One described perhaps the 'ideal-type speech therapy': 'It (speech therapy) was just right to put my speech back and then she left me alone. That is good.' The almost complete lack of suggested improvements to speech therapy resulted, it is felt, from the high rate of satisfaction and the very specific nature of the therapy.

General Comments

Respondents in the study reported marked changes in their lives due to MS and improvements in a variety of areas of functioning as a result of professional health care. These included increased physical and emotional independence and improved speech. Most benefit was achieved when the person with MS was given clear indication as to what the therapy hoped to achieve.

Perceived professional health care also clearly tied in with values held by the wider society. For example, in Australia, the USA and other highly industrialised countries, positive value is placed on possessing an occupation, being productive at a job and achieving in the labour force;[11] physical and emotional independence being highly valued, and physical attractiveness and youth also greatly emphasised.[25] The person with MS, having been socialised into these values, had clearly retained them as ideals to be achieved, despite his MS. Not surprisingly, therefore, health care professionals who were judged to help him re-achieve or retain these positive societal values were reported by him as having been the most helpful. So, physiotherapy was seen as giving physical independence and mobility, thereby offering the opportunity to improve social and sexual interaction. Speech therapy was seen as helping with social interaction by improving communication skills and self-image. Some respondents saw psychotherapy as aiding in emotional independence, improving self-image and increasing social interaction with family, staff and fellow patients— all these benefits clearly tying in with the already mentioned societal ideals.

WORK

Rehabilitation or health care, because of the nature of MS, is reported as stressing 'preserving lives and restoring human dignity', rather than 'back to work' aspects. However, even though, in Australian society, value is placed on human life and the dignity of the individual, it also supports the protestant work ethic and, with it, the value of individual independence. In the case of the person with MS, these values come into conflict.

Work in general is regarded as one of the most fundamental human activities. To be human and to work are inextricably intertwined notions,[26] so that a person's worth is measured by his work. Brewer[26] reports people as prone to describe themselves in terms of what they do and concludes that the loss of a job challenges one's very self-identity. Berger[26] reports that, for most of his history, men have been what they did. This does not mean that they have liked what they did, but it nevertheless provided a self-identification for the individual that was stable, consistent and so recognised both by others and by himself. Work, then, is valued not only for its instrumental usefulness, but also for the psychosocial side-effects which economic independence gives. It is reported as playing a crucial role in the formation of the core identity, in self-esteem, in the overall organisation of life, in family life as well as in mental health.[8, 11] Unemployment alone has been reported as causing loss of sexual drive, depression, suicide, familial disharmony, divorce, feelings of boredom and loss of financial independence.[27, 28, 29]

All people with MS in this study had lost their breadwinning capacity and, except for one who was 'waiting for a remission', none expected to return to a job. Males in particular, then, had to deal therefore not only with the marked physical and psychological stresses of MS disablement, but also, through the loss of their jobs, an attack on their 'core identity'. The female, 'non-breadwinning' people with MS continued describing themselves in terms of 'housewife' as they had done before the onset of MS. Consequently, they reported experiencing fewer disturbances in self-image, family, sex and work than did males.

The work ethic and other Australian values, although not stressed or indeed regarded as appropriate in relation to MS by most health professionals, were nevertheless basic to the reported perceptions in this study. The internalised values and norms remained, despite the crippling effects of the disease which forced most people with MS in this study into a life-style and help-seeking behaviour which were contrary to these values and norms.

STRENGTH OF SOCIETAL ATTITUDES

Societal attitudes (such as stigmatisation) and values (such as independence and work) therefore define a non-physical dimension to MS disability. The strength of societal values and the depth of their internalisation in people with MS appear at best underrated, but mostly disregarded in the rehabilitation programme. The present aim, of keeping people with MS 'physically and mentally as fit as possible for as long as possible', produces therefore a shadow system of values generally at a level well below that expected by the MS person, who still measures himself against the internalised societal ideal, and this serves to increase the sense of frustration in him. For example, he is told that he is lucky to have a supportive wife and even tries to feel lucky, till guilt feelings eventually overpower him as he realises that he is not measuring up to society's, or indeed his own, internalised values and norms. Even where a person with MS is able to stretch values and norms, he is not likely to establish a satisfactory and solid identity if he feels he still does not measure up to the socially acceptable criteria for a valid identity.

At this stage, then, the types of health care and support sought by people with MS in this study were those that tied in most with the wider society and, in doing so, restored some feelings of self-worth. However, this type of rehabilitation did cause severe frustration on the part of many persons with MS in general, and males in particular. In this regard, respondents' perceptions of the health professionals indicated that intervention was generally seen as beneficial. However, underlying their answers were strong indications that the help given to them was seen as somewhat separated from societal attitudes and was not taking internalised values into account. The outcome of this study suggests that, through further research, health professionals should become aware of the large differences in male and female perceptions of care and the fact that these perceptions are largely influenced by those societal norms and values which have been internalised by the person with MS. Therefore, if one accepts society's attitudes and the physical and mental limitations that MS places on a person, it may be important to institute research to find alternate types of health care for chronic diseases. This type of research may establish, for example, that rehabilitation, which cancels out the effects of internalised societal values and norms, may be the most appropriate and practical type for people suffering from a chronic physical disease such as MS.

SOME OPTIONS

Although the sample was small, it was felt that a number of options could be tentatively stated.

1. Some came for the cure after having 'been processed' by many doctors. This indicates that either the person received the wrong information or may have been markedly denying the reality of this illness. Both these situations have been known to occur. Some educational campaign may well be launched by the centre to keep the medical community at large up to date on the most recent findings on MS, in order to reduce these unrealistic expectations.

2. Medical services could provide a regular service whose main function would be anxiety reduction in those who feel worried about their symptoms, yet fearful that these symptoms would make them look silly if special appointments were made and no basis for these symptoms was found. Such a regular service may well be within the scope of the present medical services at the centre.

3. Nursing care might be regarded as more beneficial by patients if extra individuality were allowed in the rooms. Such extra individuality may well be possible within the centre's present structure of nursing care.

4. With occupational therapy, it would appear that more introductory information should be given at the time of induction to the centre, particularly on how occupational therapy might help the individual. The introduction of work-type programmes, including the concept of time, could be explored by the occupational therapy department, particularly in regard to males with MS. Further research into occupational therapy might find males to be more accepting of treatment if work-type activities were introduced, including the reported suggestion of structured time. Present indications are that males in particular would view such additions as making occupational therapy more helpful, particularly as they could at least partially maintain their self-image and, in particular, their core identity.

5. The reported perception that physiotherapy can make MS people feel worse should be further explored, particularly with a view to trying to develop methods in which this type of person with MS might be able to be identified earlier in the disease process.

6. Centres in general might also usefully campaign for local GPs to recommend physiotherapy earlier in the disease process of suspected and newly diagnosed people. Males, in particular, reported hoped-for benefits if this had been done for them.

7. There are indications that, in general, too much emphasis is given to physical aspects of the disease, whereas psychosocial problems appear to predominate in the disease from the point of view of the person with MS. Indications are that psychotherapeutic intervention by the centre could be usefully extended by either an increase in staff with skills in that area, or by teaching some of these skills to existing staff.

8. The centre concerned is one of the few in Australia with a speech therapist. This study indicates that this service is a valuable part of treatment, particularly for females. As a result of these perceptions and in response to their request, the centre might usefully embark on an education programme for local, general practitioners to refer those with suspected speech problems earlier to speech therapists than they have done in the past.

9. *Function of the centre*. This study indicated that another function of the centre might lie in public education in order to reduce architectural and psychosocial barriers. Problems were experienced in these areas without many of the helping professions being perceived as helpful in their solution.

Research should therefore be carried out in an attempt to find ways to diminish psychological barriers that inhibit the MS disabled from becoming integrated with 'normal' society. In this regard, it is already known that people stay at greater distances from disabled than from non-disabled persons, that they smile less, avoid eye contact and are more rigid in their body behaviour. This knowledge, however, does not appear to have influenced the care that is provided. In fact, most countries fail to include a comprehensive system of societal integration of the disabled in their rehabilitation programmes. Some countries do acknowledge the existence of prohibiting architectural barriers which interfere with the disabled, but few appear to tackle the problem effectively.

RECOMMENDATIONS

Future research, in order for planned changes to take place, should not only take cognisance of attitudes of people with MS but also relate these attitudes to the views expressed by professional staff about their efficacy and what they perceive to be successful care. Such research may raise the issue of the appropriateness of the medical model of treatment which appears to characterise most MS centres at present. In this regard, combining the results of both the interview-schedule and open-ended interview, indicates that although the centre fulfilled a number of important functions for the MS person, it appeared to leave a large number of problems untouched. It also appears that psychosocial problems in learning to cope with the illness were seen by them as being of prime importance. Although most health professionals to some extent acknowledge the importance of this, they do so largely with a curative rather than preventative orientation. The centre might serve the MS person better if it concerned itself with optimising the adaptive potential and psychosocial life skills as well as reducing the amount of physical pathology.

REFERENCES

1. Glazier W.H. (1973). The task of medicine. *Scientific American*; **228**:13.
2. Katz S. (1959). Multidisciplinary studies of illness in aged persons: a new classification of function status in activities of daily living. *Journal of Chronic Diseases*; **9**:55.
3. Albrecht G.L. (1969). Adult socialisation: the effects of aspiration and social interaction on rehabilitation. Phd dissertation. Alberta, Canada: Emory University.

4. Struening E.L., Guttentag M. (1975). *Handbook of Evaluation Research* Vol. 2. Beverly Hills: Sage Publications.
5. Ware J.E. *et al*. (1978). The measurement and meaning of patient satisfaction. *Health and Medical Care Services Review*; **1**(1):1.
6. Mechanic D. (1979). *Future Issues in Health Care*, Chapter 10. New York: Free Press.
7. Apostle D., Oder F. (1967). Factors that influence the public's view of medical care. *Journal of the American Medical Association*; **202**:572.
8. Albrecht G.L. (1976). *The Sociology of Physical Disability and Rehabilitation*. Pittsburgh: University of Pittsburgh Press.
9. Di Angelo E., Hamilton B.E., Swarts P.S., Betts H.B. (1973). Rehabilitation follow-up of the accident disabled. Unpublished manuscript held by The Rehabilitation Institute of Chicago.
10. Bergsten E., Asaba H., Bergstrom J. (1977). A study of patients on chronic haemodialysis: a sociomedical investigation of the experiences of patients on haemodialysis and their quality of life. *Scandinavian Journal of Social Medicine*; Suppl. **11**.
11. Safilios-Rothschild C. (1970). *The Sociology and Social Psychology of Disability and Rehabilitation*. New York: Random House.
12. Lilius H.E., Valtonen E.J., Wikstrom J. (1976). Sexual problems in patients suffering from multiple sclerosis. *Scandinavian Journal of Social Medicine*; **4**:41.
13. Litman T.J. (1972). Physical rehabilitation: a social–psychological approach. In *Patients, Physicians and Illness* (Jalo E.G., ed.). New York: Free Press.
14. Haber L.D. (1971). Disabling effects of chronic disease and impairment. *Journal of Chronic Diseases*; **24**:469.
15. Vas G.J. (1969). Sexual impotence and some autonomic disturbances in men with multiple sclerosis. *Acta Neurologica Scandinavica*; **45**:166.
16. Barrett M. (1981). *Sexuality and MS*. Toronto: MS Society of Canada.
17. Burnfield A., Burnfield P. (1978). Common psychological problems in multiple sclerosis. *British Medical Journal*; **1**:1193.
18. Parsons T., Fox R.C. (1968). Illness, therapy and the modern American family. In *A Modern Introduction to the Family* (Bell, W., Vogel E.F., eds.) pp. 370–90. New York: Free Press.
19. Zola I.K. (1973). Pathways to the doctor: from person to patient. *Social Science and Medicine*; **7**:677.
20. Cartwright A., Hockey L., Anderson J. (1973). *Life Before Death*. London: Routledge & Kegan Paul.
21. Fidler G., Fidler J.W. (1970). *Occupational Therapy: a Communication Process in Psychiatry*. New York: Macmillan.
22. Peach H., Pathy M.S. (1977). Evaluation of patients' assessment of Day Hospital care. *British Journal of Preventive and Social Medicine*; **31**:209.
23. Overall B., Aronson M. (1963). Expectations of psychotherapy in patients of lower socio-economic class. *American Journal of Orthopsychiatry*; **43**:41.
24. Mayer J., Timms N. (1969). Clash in perspective between worker and client.

Social Casework; January: 32.

25. Bersheid E., Walster E., Bohanstedt G. (1973). The happy American body: a survey report. *Psychology Today*; **8**:119.
26. Berger P.L. (1964). *The Human Shape of Work: Studies in the Sociology of Occupations*. Chicago: Henry Regnery.
27. Brewer G. (1975). *Workers Without Jobs: a Study of a Group of Unemployed People*. Sydney: Brotherhood of St Laurence.
28. Jahoda M., Lazersfeld P., Zeisal H. (1971). *Marienthal: The Sociography of an Unemployed Community*. Chicago: Aldine Atherton.
29. Griffiths D. (1972). *Unemployment: the Facts and Effects*. Sydney: Brotherhood of St Laurence.

Epilogue

The contributors of this book have shown that MS is not just a medical condition, but that it has many important human dimensions. Their combined effort shows that MS is a relationship between an individual and his or her environment.

Many MS societies, however, appear to overlook or not adequately care for the emotional and social sequelae of the disease in both the person with MS and his or her family. Staff composition at MS centres tends to confirm this view in that more help tends to be employed to deal with the physical and medical rather than the psychological and social aspects of the disease.

Rehabilitation and care for those people disabled with MS and their families could, however, clearly consist of a more balanced use of a combination of a variety of measures provided by medical, physical, social, psychological, educational, vocational and research staff. Furthermore, although much research in the psychological social areas is being done around the world, it has become evident that such research lacks a common bank where it can be combined and analysed for cross-cultural examination and distribution. Psychosocial research will only benefit the person with MS if it becomes more widely distributed to MS societies around the world rather than what is happening at present.

In this regard, it should be of interest to know that E. Mellerup from Denmark is researching 'the uses of family therapy' in relation to MS. B. Dick from the Swiss Society has done much work on 'couple therapy'. Troost from the Belgian Society has researched 'the effects of hospitalisation on MS-disabled people and their families'. Medaer from Belgium has written articles on, and is continuing research on, 'self-help groups and MS'. The concept of such groups is presently seen as important in relation to many disabilities.

Vocational assessment and placement have been widely researched by Rozin *et al.* in Israel and their results could clearly be of great benefit to those with MS as well as rehabilitation staff and employers.

Also, countless important research in the form of Honours, Masters and PhD theses is being lost on library shelves around the world— their contributions lost and their findings wasted.

The formation of a common 'knowledge' bank on psychological and social aspects of MS which co-ordinates and distributes such knowledge would clearly benefit many. This book, it is hoped, is the beginning of such an international effort at distributing such information to MS societies around the world.

It is also hoped that the book provides people with MS with the hope that more psychosocial understanding is being sought on the effects of MS and that such understanding will lead to a better fulfilment of their needs within rehabilitation settings as well as within the settings of their families and society.

Further Reading

GENERAL READING

Braham S., Houser H.B., Cline A., Posner M. (1975). Evaluation of the social needs of non-hospitalized chronically ill persons. 1. Study of 47 patients with multiple sclerosis. *Journal of Chronic Diseases*; **28**:401.

Davis F. (1972). *Illness, Interaction and the Self*. Belmont, Calif: Wadsworth.

Gerson E.M., Strauss A.L. (1975). Time for living: problems in chronic illness care. *Social Policy*; **6**(3):12.

Hartings M.F., Pavlov M.M., Floyd A.D. (1976). Group counselling of MS patients in a program of comprehensive care. *Journal of Chronic Diseases*; **29**:65.

Ivers R.R., Goldstein N.P. (1963), Multiple sclerosis: a current appraisal of symptoms and signs. *Proceedings of the Mayo Clinic*; **38**:457.

Johnson G.S., Johnson R.H. (1977). Social services support for multiple sclerosis patients in West of Scotland. *Lancet*; **i**:31.

Kornfeld D.S. (1972). The hospital environment: its impact on the patient. *Advances in Psychosomatic Medicine*; **8**:252.

Miles A. (1979). Some psycho-social consequences of multiple sclerosis: problems of social interaction and group identity. *British Journal of Medicine and Psychology*; **52**:321.

Miller E.J., Gwynne G.V. (1972). *A Life Apart: a Pilot Study of Residential Institutions for the Physically Handicapped and the Young Chronic Sick*. London: Tavistock.

Paulley J.W. (1976/77). Psychological management of multiple sclerosis. An overview. *Psychotherapy and Psychosomatics*; **27**:26.

Rabkin J.G., Struening E.L. (1976). Life events, stress and illness. *Science*; **194**:1013.

Stevens B.C. (1974). A pilot inquiry on the social and psychological needs of patients disabled by multiple sclerosis and other neurological diseases. *Rehabilitation*; **90**:41.

Strauss A.L., Glaser B.G. (1975). *Chronic Illness and the Quality of Life*. St Louis, Miss: C.V. Mosby.

Tittle C.R. (1972). Institutional living and rehabilitation. *Journal of Health and Social Behaviour*; **13**:263.

Wiener C.L. (1975). The burden of rheumatoid arthritis: tolerating the uncertainty. *Social Science and Medicine*; **9**:97.

FAMILY IN SOCIETY AND ITS HEALTH

Berger P.L., Kellner H. (1974). Marriage and construction of reality. In *The Family* (Coser R.L., ed.) pp. 157–74. London: Macmillan.

Crawford C.O., ed. (1971). *Health and the Family: a Medical Socialization Analysis*. New York: Macmillan.

De Witt K. (1978). The effectiveness of family therapy. *Archives of General Psychiatry*; **35**:549.

Ferber A., Mendelsohn M., Napier A. (1972). *The Book of Family Therapy*. Boston: Houghton Mifflin.

Foley V.D. (1974). *An Introduction to Family Therapy*. New York: Grune & Stratton.

Ford F.R., Herrick J. (1974). Family rules: family life styles. *American Journal of Orthopsychiatry*; **44**(1):61.

Groog S.H., Fitzgerald E.F. (1978). Subjective stress and serious illness of a spouse: wives of heart patients. *Journal of Health and Social Behaviour*; **19**:166.

Haley J. (1963). Marriage therapy. *Archives of General Psychiatry*; **8**:213.

Hoffling C., Lewis J., eds. (1980). *The Family: Evaluation and Treatment*. New York: Brunner/Mazel.

Humphreys J. (1980). Family therapy— review of outcome research. *Australian Journal of Family Therapy*; **1**:116.

Jackson J.D. (1957). The question of family homeostasis. *Psychiatry Quarterly;* **31** (Suppl.):379.

Kantor D., Lehr W. (1975). *Inside the Family: Toward a Theory of Family Process*. San Francisco: Jossey-Bass.

Livsey C.G. (1972). Physical illness and family dynamics. *Advances in Psychosomatic Medicine*; **8**:237.

Luthman S., Kirschenbaum M. (1974). *The Dynamic Family*. Palo Alto, Calif: Science and Behaviour Books.

Rounsaville B.J., Weissman M.M., Prusoff B.A. *et al.* (1979). Process of psychotherapy among depressed women with marital disputes. *American Journal of Orthopsychiatry*; **49**:505.

Skynner A.C.R. (1976). *Systems of Family and Marital Psychotherapy*. New York: Brunner/Mazel.

Slipp S., Kressell K. (1979). Difficulties in family therapy evaluation. I. A comparison of insight vs. problem solving approaches. II. Design critique recommendations. *Family Process*; **17**:409.

Stanton M.D. (1979). Drugs and the family. *Marriage and Family Review*; **2**(1):1.

Strauss M.A., (1979). Violence in the American family. *Journal of Social Issues*; **30**(2):15.

Umana R., Gross S.J., McConville M.T. (1979). *Crisis in the Family: Three Approaches*. New York: John Wiley/Gardner Press.

Wells R., Dezen A.E. (1978). The results of family therapy revisited: the non-behavioural methods. *Family Process*; **17**(3):251.

SELF-HELP PRINCIPLES AND PRACTICES

Anderson J.A.D., Buck C., Danaher K., Fry J. (1977). Users and non-users of doctors — implications for self-care. *Journal of the Royal College of General Practitioners;* **27**:155.

Borman L.D. (1976). Self-help and the professional. *Social Policy*; 7(2):46.

Gartner A., Reissman F. (1977). *Self Help in the Human Services*. San Francisco: Jossey-Bass.

Gussow A., Tracey G.S. (1976). The role of self-help clubs in adaptation to chronic illness and disability. *Social Science and Medicine*; **10**:407.

Katz A.T. (1967). Self help in rehabilitation: some theoretical aspects. *Rehabilitation Literature*; **28**:10.

Kronenfeld J.J. (1979). Self care as a panacea for the ills of the health care system: an assessment. *Social Science and Medicine*; **13A**:263.

Levin L.S. (1976). Self-care: an international perspective. *Social Policy*; 7(2):70.

Levin L.S., Katz A.H., Holst E. (1977). *Self Care*. London: Croom Helm. (A useful work on the self-help movement and consumer participation in health care delivery.)

Lorion R.P. (1976). From anecdote to research. *Social Policy*; 7(2):94.

Reissman F. (1976). The self-help movement has arrived. *Social Policy*; 7(1):63.

Robinson D, Henry S. (1977). *Self Help and Health*. London: Martin Robinson. (An important analysis of the work of self-help groups in health care delivery.)

Ross J.C. (1972). Toward a reconstruction of voluntary association theory. *British Journal of Sociology*; **23**:20.

Williamson J.D., Danaher K. (1978). *Self-care in Health*. London: Croom Helm. (An important discussion of self-help activities in self-treatment, use of fringe health practices and professional/consumer health activities.)

Wright C.R., Hyman H.H. (1958). Voluntary association membership of American adults: evidence from National Sample Surveys. *American Sociological Review*; **23**:284.

VOCATIONAL REHABILITATION, DISABILITY AND UNEMPLOYMENT

Aldes J.H. (1967). Rehabilition of multiple sclerosis patients. *Journal of Rehabilitation*; **33**(2):10.

Braham S., Houser H.B., Cline A., Posner M. (1975). Evaluation of the social needs of non-hospitalized chronically ill persons. 1. Study of 47 patients with multiple sclerosis. *Journal of Chronic Diseases*; **28**:401.

Brown E.B., (1975). Independent mobility and the disabled. In *Comprehensive Vocational Rehabilitation for Severely Disabled Persons* (Mallik K., Yuseph S., Mueller J., eds.) pp. 103–107. Washington DC: George Washington University Medical Center.

Brown J.R. (1969). Recent studies in multiple sclerosis: inferences on rehabilitation and employability. *Proceedings of the Mayo Clinic*; **44**:758.

Burk R.D. (1967). The nature of disability. *Journal of Rehabilitation*; **33**(6):10; 34.

Burk R.D. (1975). Medical characteristics of importance in determining severe disability. In *Comprehensive Vocational Rehabilitation for Severely Disabled Persons* (Mallik K., Yuseph S., Mueller J., eds.) pp.19–24. Washington DC: George Washington University Medical Center.

Christensen A., Clausen J. (1977). Social remedial measures for multiple sclerosis patients in Denmark. *Acta Neurologica Scandinavica*; **55**:394.

Fay F. (1975). Attitudinal barriers and possible solutions. In *Comprehensive Vocational Rehabilitation for Severely Disabled Persons* (Mallik K., Yuseph S., Mueller J., eds) pp. 93–8. Washington DC: George Washington University Medical Center.

Gentile F.D., Housman R.A. (1970). *Development Project in Self and Home Employment for the Handicapped*. Albertson, New York: Insurance Company of North America.

Hawkins D.E., (1975). Toward a barrier-free environment. In *Comprehensive Vocational Rehabilitation for Severely Disabled Persons* (Mallik K., Yuseph S., Mueller J., eds.) pp. 87–9. Washington DC: George Washington University Medical Center.

Heard C. (1977). Occupation role acquisition: a perspective on the chronically disabled. *American Journal of Occupational Therapy*; **31**:243.

Kelly-Hayes M. (1980). Guidelines for rehabilitation of multiple sclerosis patients. *Nursing Clinics of North America*; **15**:245.

Maher T.F. (1974). The physician and vocational rehabilitation of the disabled patient. *Journal of the Irish Medical Association*; **67**:220.

Matthews B. (1980). *Multiple Sclerosis: the Facts*. Oxford: Oxford University Press.

Noakes E.H. (1975). Breaking through the barriers to employment. In *Comprehensive Vocational Rehabilitation for Severely Disabled Persons* (Mallik K., Yuseph S., Mueller J., eds.) pp. 99–102. Washington DC: George Washington University Medical Center.

Rozin R., Schiff Y., Kahana E., Soffer D. (1975). Vocational status of multiple sclerosis patients in Israel. *Archives of Physical and Medical Rehabilitation*; **56**:300.

Schneitzer L. (1978). Rehabilitation of patients with multiple sclerosis. *Archives of Physical and Medical Rehabilitation*; **59**:430.

Towne A. (1970). Multiple sclerosis: rehabilitation, insights and outlook. *Rehabilitation Record*; **11**(6):1.

Index